A Beginner's Guide to

SPIRITUAL STUFF

and

ALTERNATIVE HEALING

SUSAN *Saliu* ✤ JAYNE *Collett*

All rights reserved; no part of this publication may be reproduced or transmitted by any means, electronic, mechanical, photocopying or otherwise, without the prior written permission of the authors – Susan Saliu and Jayne Collett.

Copyright © 2007 Susan Saliu and Jayne Collett

Second Edition
2024

ISBN 9780958072816 (Paperback)
ISBN 9781763540620 (eBook)

Saliu, Susan, 1962- .
A beginner's guide to spiritual stuff and alternative healing.

1st ed.
Bibliography.
ISBN 9780958072816 (pbk.).

1. Spiritual healing. 2. Mental healing. 3. Spiritual healing and spiritualism. 4. Spiritual life. 5. Alternative medicine. I. Collett, Jayne. II. Title.

615.852

Graphic Design, Illustrations and Cover Art by
Jayne Collett

Buy a hard copy or eBook from Amazon

The moral right of the authors has been asserted.

*For Ali, Alex, Lauren,
and my family -
the loves of my life.
Susan*

*For Carl -
I'm glad we're
in this together.
Jayne*

*A special thank you to our
beautiful sister Angela
for her help on Feng Shui.*

*And to Sheila -
Goddess. Teacher. Healer.*

Contents

Introduction	9
Metaphysical Aspects	11
Energy	19
Creating Each Moment	23
Highest Good	29
Higher Self	33
Energy Blockages	37
The Law of Attraction	39
Auras	41
Chakras	47
White Light	63
The Astral Plane	65
Yin and Yang	69
Ch'i and Meridians	73
Feng Shui	77
Death	81
Reincarnation and Past Lives	89
Karma	95
Colour	97

Psychic Phenomena: 103
- Cartomancy; Channelling; Clairaudience; Clairsentience; Clairvoyance; Dowsing; Extrasensory Perception (ESP); I Ching; Numerology; Out-of-Body Experience (OBE); Palmistry; Psychokinesis (PK); Psychometry; Runes; Scrying; Telekinesis; Telepathy

Psychic Vs Spiritual 110
Spirit Entities/Guides/Angels/Nature Spirits 113
Meditation 119
The Spiritual Stuff Wrap Up 123
Body Symbolism 125
Alternative Healing: 133
- Acupressure; Aromatherapy; Bach Flower Remedies; Australian Bush Flower Remedies; Biochemic Tissue Salts; Bowen Therapy; Breathwork and Rebirthing; Chiropractic; Crystals; Herbal Medicine; Homeopathy; Hypnotherapy; Kinesiology; Magnetic Therapy; Massage; Naturopathy; Reiki; Reflexology; Rolfing; Shiatsu; Somatic Movement; Sound Therapy; Trager; Aura, Chakra, and Spiritual Healing

Recommended Reading 155

Reference List 156

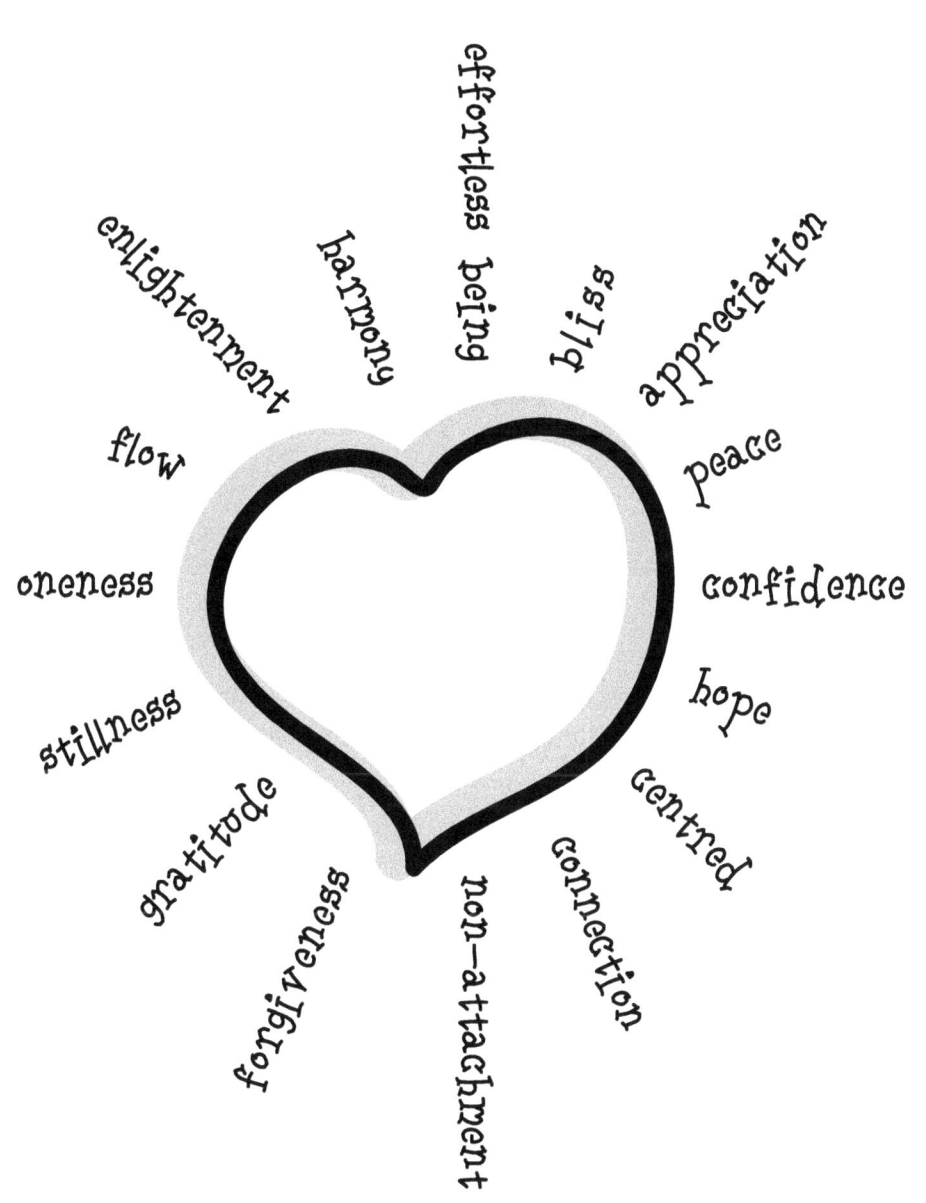

There is more to our world than meets the eye

There is a whole other world beyond it.

And everyday, in ordinary conversation with family and friends, when we would talk about this world, everyone was fascinated and interested by what we had to say. More often than not they would start asking questions –

> *"What does this mean?"*
> *"What does that mean?"*
> *"What happens when…?"*

They, too, wanted to know about this world beyond ours but they weren't prepared to read the library of books we'd read, or attend all the courses, workshops and lectures we had, just to get their questions answered. They wanted the short, sharp, shiny version.

Easy, immediate, accessible information.

So many times we tried to think of the one book we could recommend that would answer all their questions. We very quickly realised, no such book was available.

With this in mind, we created this unique guide.

It places at the fingertips of the beginner a wealth of valuable information about many of the things that are beyond our direct sensory perception; many of the things people are curious about. It introduces a wide variety of spiritual and metaphysical concepts and bathes the physical world in a new light. Even the person who has been travelling the spiritual road for a while will glean much value and insight from this work.

It can be used as an introduction guide, or as a refresher course.

As well as spiritual stuff, we've also included a run-down of some of the different methods of alternative healing which work to balance the four aspects of the self – physical, mental, emotional, spiritual.

Balance brings harmony and wellness.

Spirituality, as referred to in this guide, should not be confused with religion of any denomination. There are no divisions in spirituality. Spirituality is oneness and all things are equal – animal, vegetable and mineral.

There are as many opinions as there are people and every person will perceive the higher energies in their own way and call the higher energies whatever name feels right for them, whether it be: Allah, Buddha, God, Higher Self, Jesus, Spirit Guide, The Universe, or Vishnu, just to name a few.

We have predominantly chosen to use 'the Universe' and 'Spirit'. Please feel free to substitute your own preference.

We hope you find this guide enlightening and that you enjoy the convenience of having such diverse information within the one book.

Let your journey of discovery, creation, connection, remembering, begin.

With love and light,

Susan Saliu and Jayne Collett.

Metaphysical Aspects

The prefix 'meta',
as used in the word
metaphysical,
means:
'transcending or
going beyond'

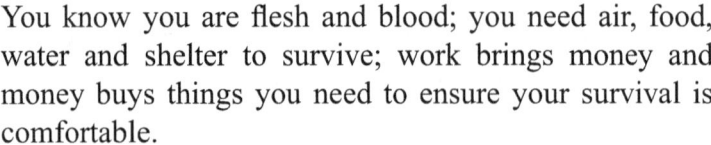

You know you are flesh and blood; you need air, food, water and shelter to survive; work brings money and money buys things you need to ensure your survival is comfortable.

You live a physical life so it's only natural that the focus of your life is on the solid world around you. What you can see and touch is real.

But, whether or not you were raised with religious or spiritual beliefs, in some way you have probably been exposed to the concept of a realm that is beyond your five senses.

Nearly every culture and society on this planet holds some kind of belief in a spiritual presence.

And it doesn't matter what you believe, chances are you've heard of:

Religion
The Aboriginal Dreamtime
The Spirit World of the Native American Indians
The Voodoo of the West Indians
Wicca

All these things, which are a few examples amongst many, are steeped in spirituality.

Additionally, mythology of Gods and Goddesses abound throughout the entire history of the world, from:

The Greek and Norse peoples
The Pagans
The Celts
The Mayans

The Druids
Buddhists
The Ancient Romans
The Egyptians
Mystical India

The suggestion of some form of a higher power is everywhere. In many instances, these higher power beliefs carry with them the further suggestion that you have a soul.

And you do have a soul.

If you already believe this, you would probably hold a personal view as to what and where your soul is.

It might also be fair to say that, more often than not, your spiritual self tends to take a backseat to your physical self because you may have been brought up to believe that you are a physical being, first and foremost, who just happens to have a soul.

However, you are more than the obvious sum of your parts:

you are actually a spiritual being, first and foremost, and a part of that energy just happens to be having a physical, human existence.

The best way to explain that statement is this - on a physical level, we have evolved over the centuries into organised societies who enjoy:

- ever-changing technology
- better medical care
- greater freedom of thought and action.

Metaphysically, your soul, or spirit, also undergoes the process of evolution but it is the *spirit* which chooses the experience of the physical existence to grow and evolve, not the other way around. To fully comprehend all facets of itself, the most effective way the soul can learn is by direct participation in relationships, events, or activities. The soul's desire for hands-on experience is why you're here on this planet.

First, we'd like to explain what we believe a soul is.

When you think about the soul you have to think beyond the length, breadth and depth of the three dimensional world you live in. This is because the energy that makes up every soul transcends the 'limited' structure of three dimensions and is not exclusively confined to this physical world.

If you 'removed' your soul from your body and stood next to it, it wouldn't look like the physical you. This is because the energy that makes up the soul does not take a rigid form and it can't be 'removed' anyway because it's everywhere: around, in, up, down and outwards - in all directions.

When you move beyond three dimensions you really have to expand your thinking to fathom the complexity of the soul energy and where that energy comes from in the first place. A common belief is that the energy that makes up each soul comes from a Source of pure, loving, highest vibrational energy.

An aspect of the energy that emanates from this Source merges with your physical self which, in turn, is an extension of Source Energy in the first place. You are a vibrational being in a vibrational universe.

Keeping in mind that your energy is not fixed conclusively, and for want of an easier way of explaining this:

Imagine your soul as being a continuous line of energy which is fastened to the Source at one end and your physical body at the other. This line of energy extends infinitely over time and space through many different energy layers.

Each layer has a particular rate of vibration so the 'section' of soul in that layer matches that rate. The vibration of the energy goes from being the highest at the Source down to the densest at the physical. This means the soul energy that is connected to your body vibrates at a lower frequency than all the energy above it. It does this to match the vibrational rate of the planet which enables you to sustain an existence at this third dimensional level.

> ***The energy is still the highest energy;***
> ***it's just buzzing a little slower.***

This continual flow of connection from the Source to you is what gives you the ability to 'feel' and 'communicate' with your spirit. By heightening your awareness about the spiritual realm you are helping to raise the vibration of your physical energy so you are better able to tune into the higher energies. You do this so you can develop a 'knowing' and a greater understanding of 'the meaning of life'.

> *Basically, the more knowledge you acquire,*
> *the 'lighter' your energy becomes.*

The aspect of your soul that exists on this physical plane is just a small part of your overall energy, like a drop of water from an ocean. This is how you stay connected to the Source at the same time as living a physical life. But know this:

*You are the Source and the Source is you.
Without the Source, there is no you.
Without you, there is no Source.
It exists because you exist. There is no separation.*

You are in partnership with your soul, not separate from it. The Source doesn't sit on high and 'expect' certain things of you so your soul can make its way back there. Your soul is already there – and here and everywhere.

Before you existed as the person you are today, your soul made a choice about what it would like to experience or, it determined which lessons to set itself.

In other words - your soul chose a life purpose and plan and set certain intentions.

It may have said something like – "I choose to know what wealth is like," or, "I choose to know what serving humanity is like," or, "I choose to learn compassion."

It can do this because soul energy is imbued with consciousness, an intelligence, and an awareness of itself. You think and feel and you accept that, but thoughts and emotions are just energy. You credit your physical brain as being the vessel that processes your thoughts yet it is a little more challenging to believe that pure energy has the same ability to process its own thoughts, but it does.

Really, there are so many things about the nature of energy we are still to learn. In the grand scheme of things most of us know about half a molecule worth of information! Imagine then all the things we don't know and haven't even thought of considering. What we don't know could quite likely fill an entire set of encyclopaedias, and more, such is the complexity of our universe.

Once your soul has established its lessons it then incarnates into the best life situation where those lessons can be most effectively learnt.

Of course your physical life will not follow such a rigidly fixed or organised plan as the soul originally set out because the probabilities, ways and means of you going about achieving your soul's purpose are innumerable. It is through the exercising of your spontaneity, free will and creative power that you can count on creating many scenarios along the way so there will be a lot of different paths from which to choose.

For the soul, it's neither here nor there whether its choices and lessons are experienced within the specified lifetime because the soul knows it has many more opportunities, in the form of other incarnations, to learn.

At first, this whole soul decision/lesson plan concept can seem highly imaginative but if you stop and think about all the situations in your life that continually pop up you will see patterns emerge. If you can reduce them down to one or two words you will have a fair idea of what you chose to gain perspective on.

To help clarify: Imagine that in all your relationships with people you end up being dominated. You feel easily intimidated and controlled but a part of you doesn't want to put up with their manipulation, yet you feel powerless to stop it. Because the situation doesn't rest easy with you, you know there is something you must do to overcome it. You must find your power and exercise it so that, in future, no one can take advantage of you.

The lesson, then, is one in strength and personal empowerment.

When you have established what your lessons are, you can make every attempt to experience them because each perspective gained raises your vibrations a little higher which then elevates your soul, bit by bit, towards a higher and higher level of consciousness and awareness.

> *The essence of the soul is pure love and hidden underneath layers of deep, physical emotions is your free and happy spirit, waiting to be found.*

Integrate your soul energy into your everyday existence. Communicate with it and use the guidance to get the best out of your life.

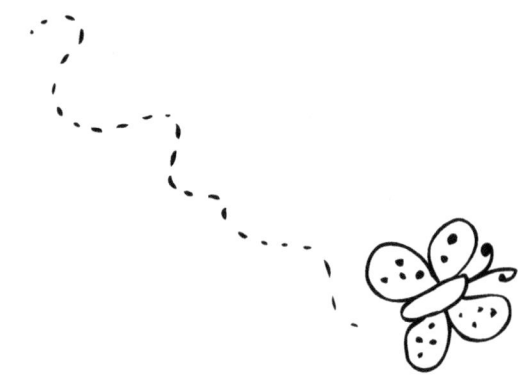

Energy

You can see now
how your physical and
metaphysical worlds
interact.

Now, let's discuss the important concept that is 'energy' in a bit more detail because it not only makes up your soul, it also makes up the whole universe around you.

When spiritual stuff and alternative healing is discussed it is common to hear things like: 'the energy of the Universe'; 'healing energy'; 'tap into the energy around you'; 'energy blockages'; 'the flow of energy'; 'channelling energy'; 'the energy of thought', plus loads more of that type of thing.

So what is this 'energy'?

Well, it's like a creative force. A force that has a vibration and an intelligence. For ease, let's compare it to the concept of love. Love is more of a feeling or a 'knowing'. It's not something you can touch or hear or see. It's not something that's tangible – it doesn't appear in physical form. You can't go and buy a box of love. Yet you know that love exists.

Spiritual energy is the same and once you consider the possibility of this energy you will begin to sense it and feel it. It will be as if you've tuned the dial on your energy radio and found the station. You will then develop your own 'knowing' about what energy is. It may not be the easiest concept to describe, but you will understand it perfectly.

Things are formed energetically before they manifest physically therefore, everything has its own energy signature. Some people can have conversations with trees and plants because their energy is resonating on the same wavelength. What you resonate with is what you will pick up on.

Energy is infinite and everywhere. It doesn't begin and end at specific points. It melds, meshes and intermingles with all other forms of energy. Even though the core essence of all energy is the same, by other forms we mean:

people energy,
tree energy,
animal, vegetable, mineral energy,
emotional energy,
thought energy.

Again, it's all the same, just resonating at different rates of vibration.

Energy is the great equaliser because each of us is made up of the exact same stuff as everyone else - from the richest person to the poorest; from the most famous to the completely unknown.

The things that make us appear different are only the physical attributes we possess – hair/eye/skin colour, height and weight, plus our individual skills, interests and talents.

In metaphysics, energy takes many forms, is channelled to you via lots of different means and can be utilised by you in many different ways.

When it all boils down to it, regardless of its classification, energy is energy.

The energy which surrounds you, inside and out, issues forth from the one Source. Everything physical was spiritual energy first.

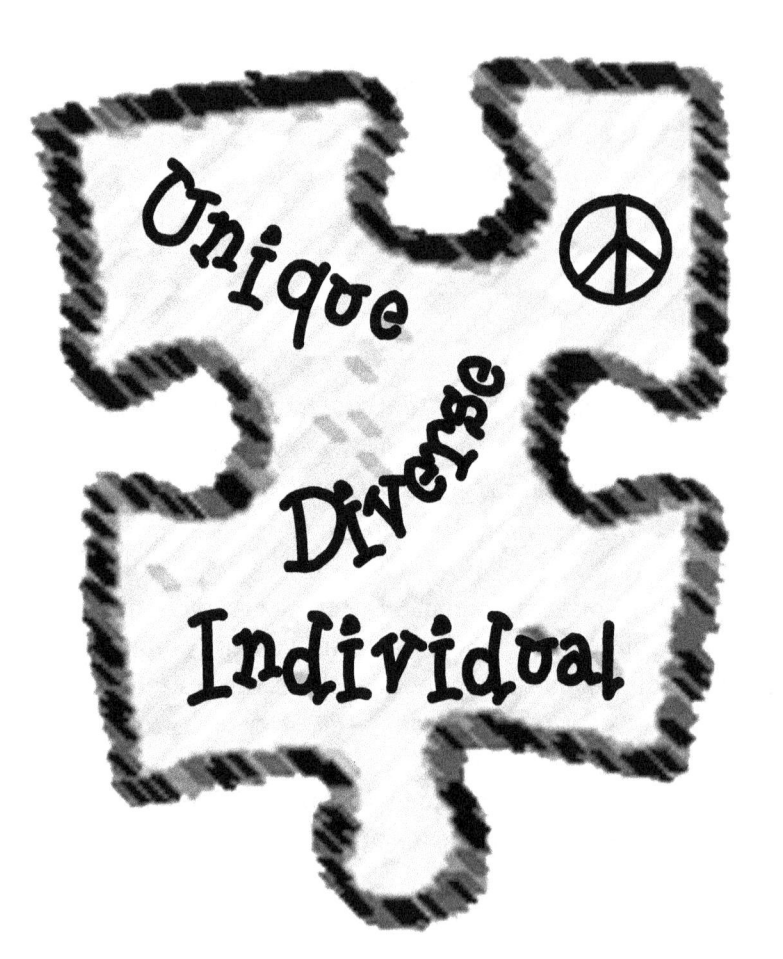

Creating Each Moment

The desire
of every spirit
is to grow,
evolve and
create.

To create is to bring something into being and each moment of your life is an expression of who you are.

Your thoughts, feelings, words and actions lead to choices and decisions which bring about specific results, and those results are the moments you find yourself living.

You can purchase a set of ingredients to create a meal, for instance, and how you put those ingredients together determines what you get. Life is very much like that.

You are in charge of creating your own life for several reasons:

- you can set up personal situations for your lessons
- the conscious and unconscious choices and decisions you make often highlight things in your life that need your attention
- you are always teaching yourself something because your spirit desires to create, experience, feel and understand.

✱Setting up lessons✱

When we refer to lessons we're talking about the various things your spirit has intended to specifically experience in a particular lifetime in order to grow and evolve.

The lessons you choose for yourself before you incarnate become important as you make your way through your life. An aspect of your energy holds the knowledge of your lesson choices and some of the decisions you find yourself making will be based on what your spirit chose to learn.

We said earlier that the soul isn't too bothered if a lesson is learnt or not because its opportunities for growth and evolvement are plentiful, but that's not to say you don't at least set yourself up to try. You will always make an attempt to learn your lessons. Your intuition is often your guide to this, as are the patterns of your life that continually repeat themselves.

You are a spiritual being living in a physical world and with that comes free will. Because of this, you are free to make choices that completely defy the intuitive urging of your spirit. You either heed your instincts or you don't.

Choices and options are available to you at every turn and the moments that make up your life are a working union of body and soul.

> *The things you do in the physical will be influenced by the spiritual.*
>
> *The things you achieve on a spiritual level will be influenced by the physical.*

✸ *Things that need your attention* ✸

As you live your life you are not conscious that you are creating it moment by moment. It's just something that is. Every now and then though, something will crop up that needs your attention.

> ***And your attention is required because there is something important to be learnt.***

Your personal thoughts, attitudes and actions all contribute to how your days look and the simplest and most sure-fire way to recognise what needs your attention is to learn to notice repeat thoughts and repeat patterns of behaviour - all the 'same stuff, different day' things. Notice all the ways in which you wish things were different. Notice what makes you feel good and what makes you feel bad. Notice where your passions lie and notice where and why those desires aren't being met. Notice where you keep on making the same 'mistakes' or the same 'bad' decisions.

Be as objective as you can.

Try and stand outside of yourself and view your life in the third person. What would you say about it? What would you notice? Observing your creations and noticing repeat thoughts and patterns is so important because it's an effective way of highlighting the things that need your attention. Perhaps you've been ignoring your intuition? Perhaps you 'know' or 'feel' that you should be doing something particular but that gets ignored too. Repetition is akin to a spiritual message and if you don't listen – you will be shown!

Listening to your inner dialogue,
paying attention to your outer world,
actively observing your life,
and following your guidance
are all ways of communicating with Spirit.

✹ *Teaching yourself* ✹

A big part of your life is about learning and experiencing things and the knowledge you gain through observing your creations can teach you so much about yourself.

Each choice you make has a profound influence on every moment of your being.

Each individual journey is an intensely personal one and you are the master of your own destiny. You alone are responsible for the details of the trip.

It's up to you what your life is and, being a creator, you have the power - moment to moment - to make new choices. Discovering this power is discovering your spirit.

Look at your life and consider: What do your choices teach you about yourself? Are the moments you are creating joyful and fulfilling? Is your life peaceful to live? What do you want your moments to be filled with? What do you deserve to have in your life? What is your passion? What excites you?

There will be key moments in your life where Spirit will work closely with you to remind you of your lessons; to guide you towards a particular path which aligns with your soul purpose this lifetime. The rest of your life is up to you. The thoughts you think, the words you speak, the actions you decide to take, or not take, all contribute towards your creation.

*Thoughts. Words. Actions.
Desire. Inspiration. Intention. Expectations.
Feelings. Emotions. Attitude. Perception.
Conscious and Subconscious Beliefs.
These are your palette and your life is your canvas.*

Just as an artist creates a unique and individual piece of work, you too have the same abilities to produce moment by moment masterpieces.

Use this gift of creation well.

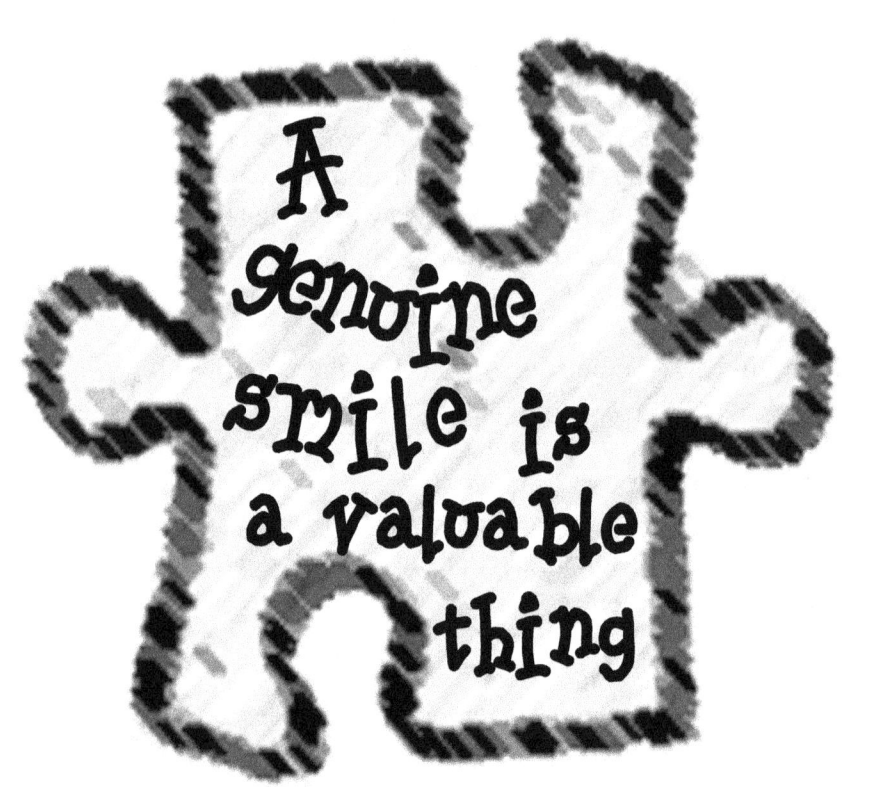

Highest Good

The term
'Highest Good'
refers to what is good
and right for your soul
as opposed to what you
would like to think is
good and right for
your physical self.

Say you really wanted a particular job and you asked the Universe to help you secure it.

You believe it'll be the best thing that's ever happened to you. It's your area of expertise. You'll work overtime, go on a health kick, give up sugar, etc. Whatever it takes, you'll do it. You really, really want this job.

And after all that bargaining and hope, you don't get it.

It would be so easy to feel cheated and disappointed and let down.

But, believe it or not, the outcome was perfect.

What happened is that, in keeping with the intentions, lessons and evolution of your soul, the outcome was for your highest good.

You won't know all the intricacies of the lessons you chose to learn but you can trust that the Universe is always working with you.

The essence of the Universe is well-being.

Maybe something better turns up a few weeks later or maybe you needed to be in a particular place on a particular day for a significant, life-changing event to occur and if you had been working in that job it wouldn't have been possible.

The outcome of certain situations and events in your life may not always thrill you but everything happens for a reason and your life is working perfectly.

Frustrating as that can seem at times, your soul energy is always aligned with its purpose. Spiritually, something gets achieved.

The exact same principle applies for events that affect life on a global scale, such as natural disasters or war. Even though it may not always be immediately obvious, whatever happens and whatever the results are, it is always for the highest good of the planet.

So much progress, growth, evolvement and change occurs quickly when 'big' things happen in the world.

Keep on asking the higher forces for the things you desire but instead of seeking a specific outcome, ask instead that the outcome be for your highest good.

**You don't need to guide the Universe.
The Universe will guide you.**

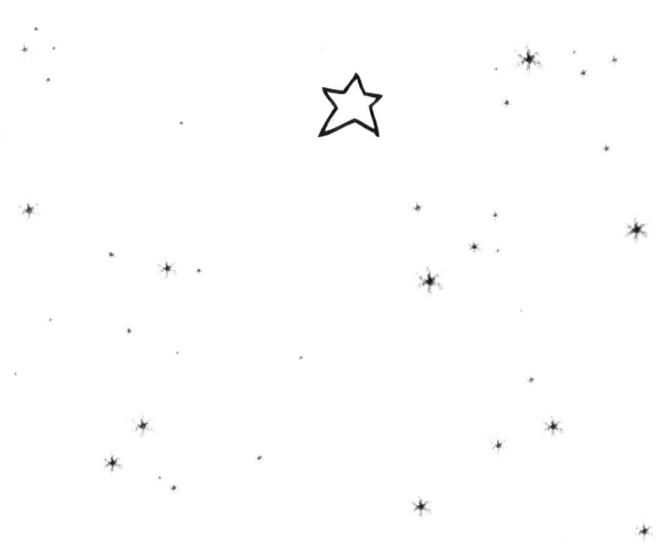

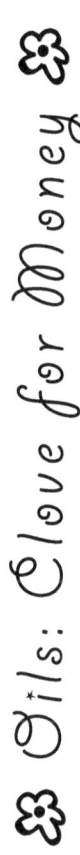

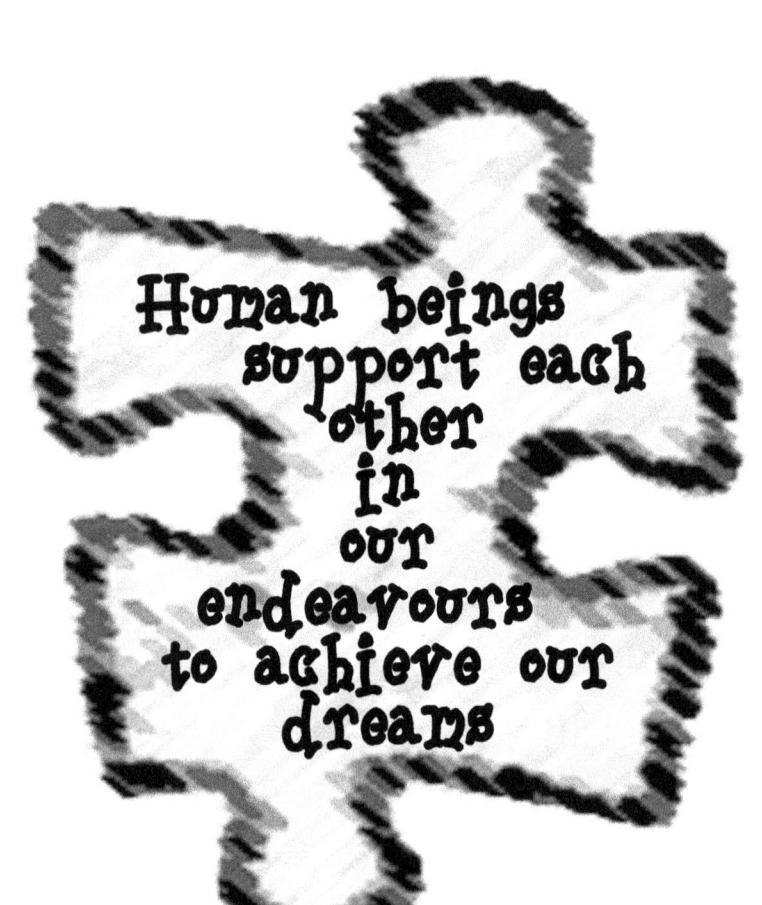

Higher Self

'Higher Self' is a term used to refer to an aspect of yourself that is not physically incarnated. It is a very real part of your energy but it is not 'visible' to the untrained, naked eye.

Your higher self knows every single thing about you. It knows what you need for your spiritual and physical growth and evolvement. It knows the blue print for your life on Earth.

It holds the knowledge of the life lessons you chose to experience and it knows what choices you will make before you make them.

Instinctive feelings and thoughts filter through to you from your higher self. Have you ever just known something but you're not sure how you knew it? Have you ever had a stray thought pop into your head and you're not sure where it came from? That's your higher self communicating with your physical self, providing you with guidance.

The saying 'follow your instincts' did not come about by accident.

If you learn to tune into your higher voice you will have the answers you seek, that are right for you and appropriate to your growth, when you seek them.

Your higher self also communicates with the higher self of others. They make plans to orchestrate appropriate movements and proceedings that will result in definitive actions.

Whether your physical self acts upon these plans is entirely up to you. Your higher self would never 'make' you do anything which is contrary to your growth or anything that does not serve your best interests.

The higher self is pure love and, because it does not hold

'physical' emotions, it does not judge or act with malicious intent.

All guidance is always for the highest good of the individual.

You've heard of being in the right place at the right time or you've marvelled at how perfectly things worked out in a given moment that resulted in some life changing event. These things are no accident. These things are in front of your nose so you can not only learn something but so you can think about how such things came to be and the forces that 'made' them be.

Coincidences, or more accurately, co-incidences, exist.

They are events orchestrated in co-operation with yourself and other energies. Think about a co-incidence in your life, break it down into parts and see how every piece fitted another perfectly, like a jigsaw, until the whole picture was complete. You'll be surprised at the precision of play and the 'perfection' of every moment.

Don't discount what you can't see.

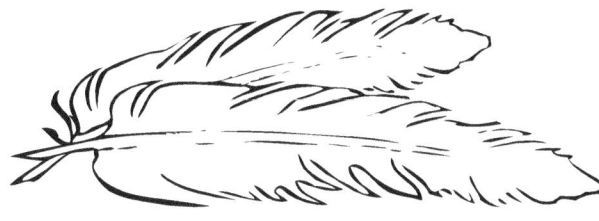

When I support others, I support myself

Energy Blockages

Blocked energies are old energies that have, for want of a better analogy, formed themselves into stagnant, resistant masses inside you.

You inadvertently allow energy blockages to form because you swallow, deny, stuff and hold down your emotions instead of expressing them, which allows them to be released from your body.

Every time you've felt powerless, traumatised, hurt, rejected, neglected, betrayed, inconsequential, inadequate, intimidated, failed to stand up for yourself, or failed to express your feelings to those who you felt had hurt you, your energy 'glued' up.

Exactly where the energy stopped flowing freely would depend on the emotion that was never released.

*If you didn't express anger, for instance,
an energy block may have formed in your liver.*

These hurts can go as far back as a harsh word or action you encountered in your childhood.

Each emotion that goes unexpressed eventually leads to the 'glue' getting so thick that energy has difficulty flowing through the sticky mess, either in or out.

Energy blocks often result in physical and mental illness because old, rancid emotions in your body, like open wounds, eventually fester and thus create maladies and ailments.

✧See 'Ch'i and Meridians' and 'Body Symbolism' for further organ/emotion correlations✧

I am aligned with my purpose

The Law of Attraction

The Law of Attraction
is a Universal law
that says
'like attracts like'.

The law tells us the energy of your thoughts and feelings and beliefs are like magnets - the things you think about, focus on, expect to happen, have strong feelings about, are what you attract into your space.

For instance, happy attracts situations of happiness, fear attracts situations that cause worry and dread, positive thinking attracts positive outcomes, etc.

The stronger the feeling that goes with the thought, the more powerful the 'attraction' vibration of the energy.

The Law of Attraction can be applied to your physical, mental, emotional and spiritual self.

You can attract material possessions, change your life situations so you're happy and content, and gain an understanding of who you are and what you want.

Essentially, you can attract your way to a personally satisfying life.

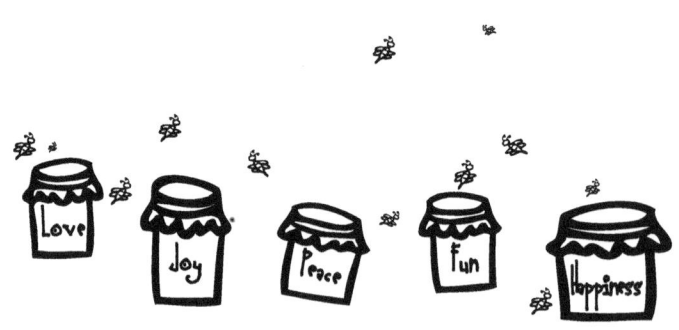

Aura

The human aura is a
multi-coloured and
multi-layered energy
field that surrounds
the physical body and
can be sensed, or seen,
by someone who
is in tune with the
energies around them.

It is generally accepted that there are seven layers of the aura, each of which contains information about your physical, emotional, mental and spiritual state and are distinctive from one another in appearance and function.

The energies of your aura are sensitive to each and every one of your emotions and by assessing the clarity of the hues, your level of health can be revealed.

It is considered that bright, radiant colours are indicative of good health whilst discoloured, smeary colours suggest imbalance or illness.

A person who can read auras would be able to detect an impending illness before it manifested itself into the physical body because your highly responsive energies are affected before your body is.

Early detection and cleansing of any auric deficiencies could help prevent a physical illness from taking hold.

Much information has been written about the aura but the names and descriptions given below are based on those sensed by Barbara Ann Brennan and written about in her book '*Hands of Light*', (Bantam Books, 1987).

From first to seventh, the layers are as follows:

THE ETHERIC BODY: The term 'etheric' is derived from the word 'ether' which, in Greek Mythology, was believed to be the element which made up all heavenly bodies. The etheric layer hugs the physical body, exactly replicating its structure and anatomy. Energetically it extends anywhere from half a centimetre up to five centimetres from the body. The colour varies from light blue to grey.

THE EMOTIONAL BODY: As its name indicates, this layer deals with your emotions - how you feel about yourself and others, and pertains to your emotional psychology in general. Love, anger, joy, hate, stress, etc., affect the energy of this layer. The emotional body is made up of swirling, flowing masses of multi-coloured clouds which extend two to eight centimetres from the body. Because the energy changes and moves, the shape of the emotional body is less defined than the etheric and bears only an approximate resemblance to that of the physical.

THE MENTAL BODY: Extending from eight to twenty centimetres from the body, yellow in colour and progressively less defined than the previous two layers, the mental body is associated with mental processes, ideas and thoughts. Because of the nature of the layer, it tends to be most visible around the head and shoulders. Concentrating on a task, or thinking hard about something, expands the energy further outwards. It also becomes brighter.

THE ASTRAL BODY: Similar in composition to the emotional body, the astral body has no definite form or distinct shape and likewise consists of multi-coloured clouds which respond to the psychology of the person. This auric layer is associated with love and relationships and it is here where strong, emotional bonds are formed. It extends out about fifteen to thirty centimetres from the body. The astral body is the fourth and middle layer of the aura.

THE ETHERIC TEMPLATE BODY: A template is a pattern or gauge which is used as a guide to reproduce shapes accurately. The etheric template acts as such a guide and it is from this fifth layer of the aura that the first layer takes its form. Should the etheric layer be damaged in any way, when healing work is done the template is 'used' to restore it to its original state. The energy of the template body resonates at a higher rate than that of its copy so an imbalance would show up as a disturbance in the vibrations of the energy, rather than as changes to its deep blue colour. It is said to be eggshell shaped and extends forty five to sixty centimetres from the physical body.

THE CELESTIAL BODY: Streams of soft, multi-coloured light, set in no particular shape, which glow radiantly from the centre of the body, make up this spiritually emotional layer of the aura. Extending about sixty to eighty centimetres from the body, it is through this layer you become aware of your connection to Spirit and are able to open up the channels of communication. You also experience unconditional love and trust.

THE KETHERIC TEMPLATE: Also known as the Causal Body, is the spiritually mental layer of the aura. With an extension of seventy five to one hundred centimetres around the body, it is through this golden layer you can become one with Spirit. Through the ketheric level, which holds your life plan, you can study your past lives.

In addition to the above, the energy of your aura is extremely sensitive to other energies around it.

Have you ever felt uncomfortable if someone stood too close to you or you just didn't like someone on sight, but you couldn't quite explain why? That's your aura picking up the energy from their aura and letting you know that their energy is not compatible with yours, for whatever reason that might be.

Having your space invaded is a very real thing and it's not

just your physical body that finds it hard to cope with, it's your aura first.

In many respects the aura is the first line of defence when it comes to warning you about a situation. Just as a cat's whiskers act as sensors so the animal can avoid endangering itself, your aura helps you in the same way.

***Trust your instincts if your
comfort zone is being compromised.***

***Energy 'knows' immediately what it
sometimes takes you a while to figure out.***

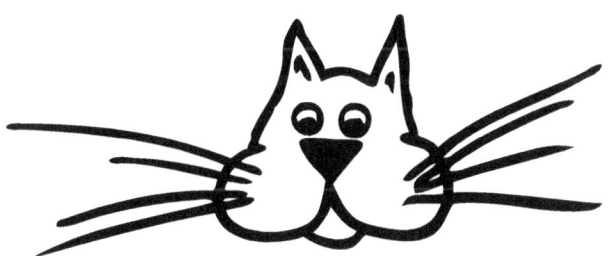

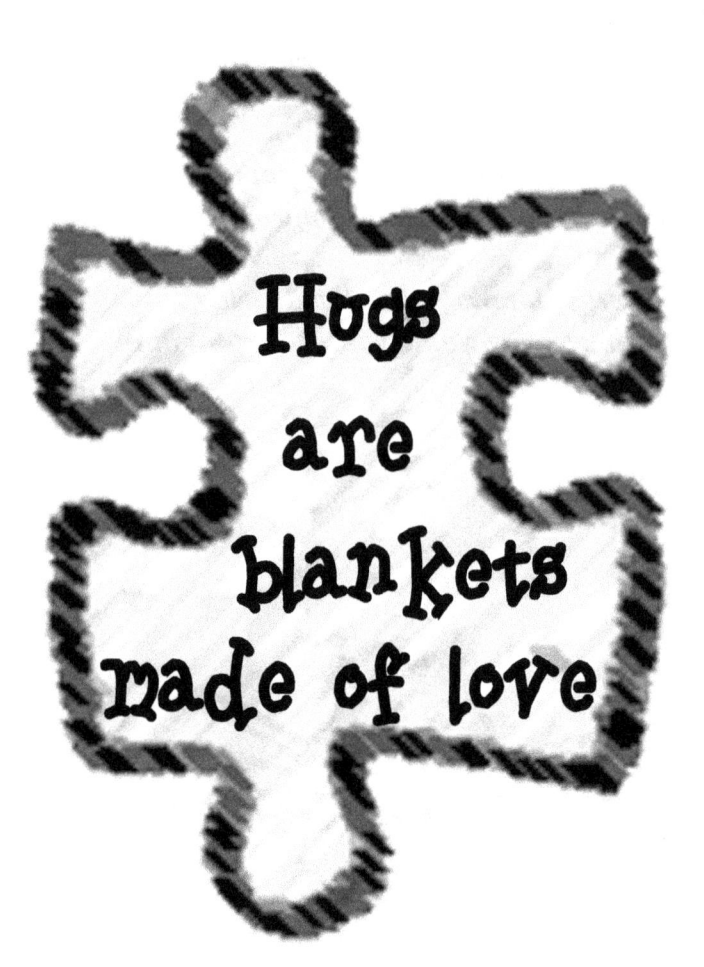

Chakras

The word Chakra
comes from the Sanskrit,
an ancient language of
India now only used for
religious purposes,
and means 'wheel'.

Chakras are swirling energy centres, or vortexes, located at specific points within, and extending outside of, your body. You have many chakras but, to keep things uncomplicated, we'll focus on seven main charkas which are positioned in the centre of your body following the line of the backbone, starting at the base of the spine and finishing at the crown of the head.

The basic job of each chakra is to act as an agent for life-force energy coming into the body, helping to distribute it throughout.

The position and colour of the chakra determines its specific spiritual, emotional, mental and physical function.

As the subject of chakras can be very involved, we're going to present them here according to Western tradition which widely accepts that the colours of the seven main chakras correspond to the seven colours of the rainbow.

But, in effect, each chakra contains all the colours of the other chakras and therefore variances in colour may be sensed. There is no hard and fast rule. Remember, go with what you feel.

The seven main chakras are:

B̲a̲s̲e̲/R̲o̲o̲t̲ – the base, or root, chakra is **red** and can be found at the base of the spine, in line with the genitalia. Red is a 'hot', energising colour and is suitable for provoking activity. The intense heat red depicts provides you with the necessary energy, strength, passion, courage, stimulation, vitality and assertiveness needed to survive in this physical world.

The energy of the base chakra concerns itself primarily with security and support, especially that which comes from your family. From birth, you have basic biological and psychological needs. These needs include food, shelter and nurturing.

If these needs are satisfied, you feel safe and secure within yourself and develop a sense of emotional and mental stability which enables you to move forward in your life.

If these needs aren't met you tend to spend a lot of your time, as you get older, trying to satisfy what you missed out on.

Unlike the other chakras, which generate their energy outwards from the body, the base chakra points down towards the earth, connecting you firmly to the physical.

This anchor keeps you grounded, i.e. your feet firmly on the ground, and enables you to achieve the necessary skills to survive whilst you live on the Earth plane. Being grounded allows you to be centred and focused so you are able to deal with the day to day aspects of life and it ensures you are fully participating in being of this world and experiencing the necessary emotions which are vital for your spiritual growth.

The glands and organs affected by the base chakra are the adrenals, colon, legs, spinal column, bones.

Suitable crystals to help heal and energise the base chakra are Bloodstone or Black Onyx.

**What images does the colour red invoke for you?
Do you need more, or less, red in your life?**

SACRAL – the sacral chakra is **orange** and located in the centre of the area between the base chakra and the belly button. Being a slightly cooler colour than red it is, nevertheless, still very warm but it lacks the impulsiveness that red represents, instead, making you think before you act, although the action will probably be inspired by enthusiasm rather than logic because it provides a balance between the impetuousness of the base chakra and the rationalism associated with the yellow of the solar plexus chakra.

The colour orange inspires imagination, optimism, adaptability and encouragement because it is such an uplifting, enlivening colour.

Sacral chakra energy concerns itself with personal power, creativity, sexuality and relationships.

Personality wise, everyone is different so it is the job of your sacral chakra energy to let you know who you truly are. It reminds you that you have the potential to be and do what you desire, whilst respecting those around you at the same time.

It reminds you that you don't have to continually conform or comply just to be accepted.

It helps you establish a strong sense of personal power so you can feel secure in the certainty that you have the right to make choices.

It is about integrity in your relationships - honesty and mutual respect, and it is about bonding with others who support your growth and development and releasing those relationships you find repressive.

It is about being comfortable with sex and sexuality, so no judgements about yourself, or others, are made.

Sacral chakra energy also aids in bringing your creative ideas to fruition.

*The organs affected by the sacral chakra are those contained within the pelvic girdle –
the internal reproductive organs, bladder,
lower portion of the intestines and the rectum.*

Suitable crystals to use are Amber or Topaz.

**What does the colour orange arouse in you?
When are you most drawn to the colour orange?**

S<small>OLAR</small> P<small>LEXUS</small> – the solar plexus chakra is **yellow** and can be found half a hand width above the navel. A warm colour, the brightness of yellow is joyful and stimulating and is representative of learning, harmony and coping with changes. It is the colour of the intellect. The solar plexus area is the seat of your emotions and the third chakra energy embodies your levels of self-esteem, self-worth, self-respect, self-acceptance and personal empowerment.

*The energy of the solar plexus chakra
concerns itself with you accepting yourself
as you are, building on your inner strengths,
being comfortable in your skin and
confident about your choices.*

It's about standing firm in your beliefs; taking risks and trying new things, rather than adhering to what's safe, and then taking responsibility for your choices.

Oils: Cinnamon for Psychic Awareness

A balanced solar plexus chakra allows you to reach a level of ease and comfort with who you are and your ability to stand on your own and take charge.

Knowing that you are complete, perfect and special is your divine birthright.

Health wise, the glands and organs affected by the solar plexus chakra are the pancreas, adrenals, stomach, liver, gall bladder and nervous system.

Suitable crystals to use are Citrine and Tiger's Eye.

What feelings does the colour yellow stir in you?
What part does the colour yellow play in your life?

The three lower chakras are 'hot' colours and the emotions relevant to them are 'hot' ones. Personal and family matters relating to survival, who you are and how you are perceived by others are important, highly emotional issues.

First and foremost, a strong sense of family is the foundation which gives you a basis of belonging. Because you rely so heavily on family support to survive, until you're fully self-sufficient and can support yourself, the importance family plays and how their support, or lack of it, can affect you is established very early on in life. Making your way in the world, your relationships with others and achieving what you desire will determine your level of happiness, satisfaction and fulfilment.

The concept of 'family' eventually extends beyond your

bloodline to include your community, city, state and country until it goes all the way around to embrace all of humankind. How you feel and act beyond the confines of your immediate family is largely dependant on habits and thought patterns formed during your impressionable years.

Keeping the energy balanced and flowing in these chakras allows you to be confident in all aspects of your social and personal self.

As you travel upwards from your lower charkas you begin to move away from the strong pull of your physical life. The next energy centre is the heart chakra and, being the middle one, it is here where you begin your progression towards the spiritual realms and to an understanding of your innate divinity.

<u>Heart</u> – the heart chakra combines elements of both the physical and the spiritual and is located in the centre of the chest. Its colour is **green**. Green, a combination of yellow and blue, is cool, soothing and calming and is accepted as being the colour of luck, harmony, cleansing, balance and changing direction or attitudes. Green, being a prevalent colour of nature, naturally brings about feelings of peace.

This energy centre concerns itself with love, compassion, acceptance and forgiveness, of self and others.

The heart is the predominant chakra that aids in the transition from an existence that is purely physical, to one which incorporates the importance of the spiritual and higher consciousness.

While the three lower chakras deal with your external world, your heart chakra helps you to deal with, and understand, your inner emotional world. You begin to ask yourself:

> *Do I acknowledge my emotional needs?*
> *Do I understand my emotional responses?*
> *Do I come from a place of love and empathy?*
> *Am I in touch with my deepest feelings?*

Such questions show that you must seriously acknowledge the part you play in your own life. You begin to realise that the only individual controlling your choices and destiny is yourself. Not your parents or partner. Not your children or employer. Not the television or newspapers and not 'society'.

> **You are a stand alone individual and**
> **you must acknowledge that.**

When you realise you are in charge of yourself and your emotions, you become empowered and accountable. No alibis; no escape.

There is a saying that you must love yourself before you can truly love another.

> *To love yourself is to know you are*
> *valuable, sacred and important.*

> *To love yourself is to be true to*
> *yourself and to honour yourself.*

The energy of your heart chakra encourages
you to love yourself first and foremost.

Additionally, your heart chakra encourages you to share your life with others and enjoy the feelings of love those connections bring. It also deals with love on an intimate level. Merging your energy with another is one of the finest feelings in the world. To envelop yourself in someone else's warmth and love is truly divine. Does anything else compare?

Heart chakra energy helps you get in touch with your true feelings. Love for oneself and all others which knows no negativity is the very essence of your spiritual nature.

The glands and organs the heart chakra concerns itself with are the heart, thymus, circulatory system, arms, hands and lungs.

The colour **pink** is also associated with this chakra but its focus is directed to self-love. Pink encourages self-nurturing and also pertains to honour, morality and friendships.

Crystals for the heart chakra - Jade and Rose Quartz.

**How does the colour green make you feel?
What do you love about the colour pink?**

T<small>HROAT</small> – the throat chakra is **blue** and found where its name suggests. Blue is a cool, soothing, healing colour. Energetically, this chakra is concerned with self-expression and communication; about speaking ones own truth.

The throat is also the willpower chakra and its lessons are about accepting the consequences of your choices and taking personal responsibility for your decisions.

Speaking up and saying what you really feel can be very difficult. Many things may stop you:

- You're scared of hurting feelings.
- You're worried you'll be misunderstood.
- You don't quite know how to say it.
- You are so conditioned not to speak, you can't undo its hold.
- You feel that some things are better left unsaid.
- You don't know how to say it nicely.

Words can cut like a knife and once they've been said, nothing can take them back.

Fortunately, the blue of the throat chakra aids you with your ability to speak your truths in a calm, controlled and loving manner; to express yourself honestly and openly.

Spiritually, your throat chakra is in tune with the energies of the Universe on a greater level than the four chakras below it.

The glands and organs affected by the throat chakra are the thyroid, parathyroid, throat, mouth and hypothalamus.

Healing crystals include Lapis Lazuli and Blue Lace Agate.

What does the colour blue make you want to express? How many times have you been silenced?

THIRD EYE/BROW – located in the centre of the forehead, the third eye chakra is the colour **indigo**. Indigo is associated with imagination, meditation and spirit communication. It is a cooling and purifying colour and one which promotes clarity. It is also considered to be a psychic colour.

Physically, this chakra deals with the mind - your intellect, intelligence and wisdom. Metaphysically, the energy of this chakra activates intuition, inspiration and inner vision.

Most people have heard about the 'third eye'. Interestingly, most people accept it as a truth, even though it can't be seen. This could be because the third eye energy is too strong to ignore. For all the things we don't want to believe, we give this chakra the benefit of the doubt.

This indicates that it is our innate desire to be as one with the energies around us.

This energy allows you to trust your instincts and follow your inner guidance with discernment and clarity of mind. This chakra is the proof positive that there is 'something else out there'. Have you ever had an inexplicably strong urge to do something for no apparent reason, like make a phone call or visit someone only to discover they were in distress and needing your help? Or perhaps they were just thinking about you and wondering how you were?

Don't fob off these kinds of occurrences as lucky accidents.

Expand your thinking to accept that something other than chance was at play here. Once you begin to accept these signs, you will notice they happen much more frequently.

Listen to your inner voice. It gives you information for a reason.

*The glands and organs ruled by the third eye chakra
are the pituitary gland, nose, ears and eyes.*

*Wonderful crystals for enhancing third eye properties
are Amethyst and Sodalite.*

**Close your eyes and visualise the colour indigo.
What do you experience?
What do you sense?**

CROWN – the crown chakra is **violet** and is found at the top of the head. Violet is the colour of self-improvement, peace and inspiration. It is also a powerful healing and purifying colour. This chakra connects you to your spiritual self. It is aligned to the energies of devotion, selflessness, inspiration and mysticism. Universal life force energy flows through your crown chakra and is distributed throughout all your systems. It is a gateway for healing energies and spiritual guidance.

**Through this chakra you establish a connection
with the Divine, as you perceive it, and you
reach a point of surrender and faith
with a higher power.**

Really, by the time you've unblocked, re-energised and thoroughly cleansed your other chakras and worked your way to the top of our head, you're in a pretty good way physically, mentally, emotionally and spiritually.

You've accepted that life is more than what you see.

You have faith that your life is being played out exactly as it should.

You don't worry, because there's nothing to worry about. You operate from a place of love and you see that everything on this planet is equal - animal, vegetable and mineral.

You don't judge and you trust implicitly that all is well, that the Universe will always provide for you and that you are on the right path for your soul's journey.

You are relaxed, happy and content.

You know that things 'are what they are' and 'what is – just is'.

You go with the flow, never against it.

Can you imagine living full-time with this attitude?

How easy every day would be. You'd get out of bed, thrilled to face the new day knowing that you're wrapped in a permanent coat of protective, spiritual energy. Problems would be quickly and easily resolved. Your love and peace energies would be like a magnet, attracting anyone who needed a feel-good boost. People would love to be around you and you would love to be around them. Everything you did would be because you wanted to do it, not because you had to. You would know total freedom. No self-imposed chains, burdens, or obligations.

Your soul doesn't want you to sweat the small stuff.

Your soul knows that you waste too much energy on trivialities. When you open up your crown, you open up possibilities. You tap into a universe full of wisdom. You open up a better way of life. You open up an endless supply of peace.

People dream of such peace. They pay thousands of dollars going to island resorts in the hope of achieving a semblance of it yet we can all have it, all the time. Getting there is both challenging and rewarding.

Your soul wants you to know it, as it knows you.

The gland associated with the crown chakra is the pineal gland.

The philosopher René Descartes – "I think, therefore I am" – was of the belief that the pineal gland housed the 'mind'.

Crystals for the crown are Clear Quartz and Sugalite.

What does the colour violet inspire you to do? How much energy do you waste sweating the small stuff?

ஃ

Your upper energies concern themselves less with how you interact with others and more how you interact with your personal self. How others think and feel about you becomes secondary to how you think and feel about yourself.

Through the four higher chakras you begin to learn where your personal strengths and weaknesses are and you start to work on creating a life of peace, happiness and blessed contentment. You desire only to move forward. You want what's best for yourself and you know you are the only one responsible for how your life is panning out.

The three lower chakras teach you how to deal with the world and to accept that you need to experience certain things in order to ascend to the higher vibrational, spiritual levels.

The upper chakras are cooler colours which tell you that the 'fight for survival' frictions which help to create the heat of the lower chakras are not necessary for your spiritual growth because:

Enlightenment is achieved lightly.

The cooler colours remind you to stay calm; to keep an open heart and an open mind.

You teach others how they too can take control of their lives and you do it without compromise, expectation, judgement, or ego. You become the model and example they desire to emulate. You embody all the best aspects of the human being:

You love well.
You speak well.
You heed your intuition.
You trust.

✧In the section on Alternative Healing, we'll look at why the aura and chakras may become blocked and how they can be healed and balanced✧

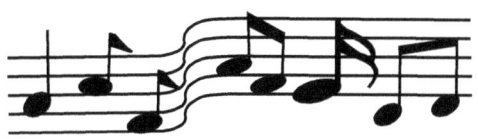

CHAKRAS

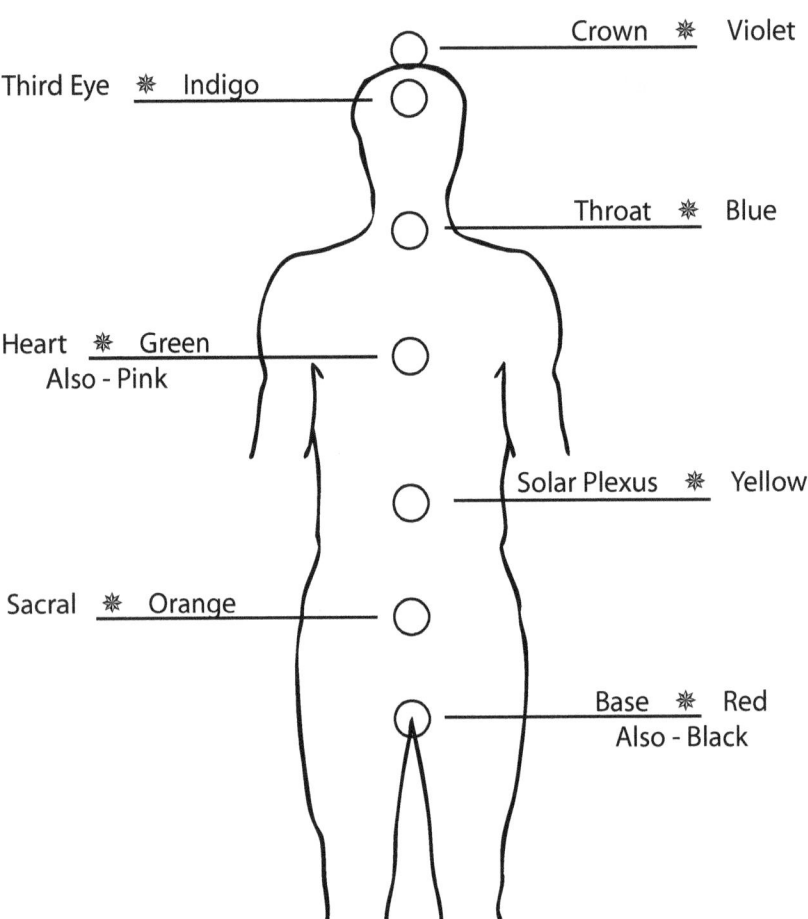

White Light

Is a term which refers to the energy that comes to you from the highest spiritual realm and is an energy you can call upon and use in many ways.

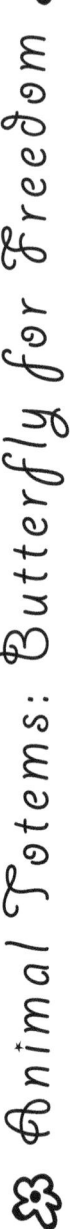

When you call upon the white light energy you set an intention for the purpose in which you would like to use it, namely - cleansing, healing, protection, meditation.

White light is a pure, loving, peaceful energy and you can ask it to flow over and through you and work with your energy systems and your physical body to cleanse, uplift and purify at the same time as raising the vibrations of your 'denser' energies so you are better able to connect to your higher energies.

You can focus on drawing white light into and around your aura to use as a source of protection.

White light contains all the colours of the spectrum and, spiritually, the colour white personifies perfection and wholeness.

Because of the high vibrational nature of the white light energy it can act as a protective shield so you can white light your houses, cars, pets, children and anything you desire to protect.

To call in the White Light say:

'In the name of the Universe I ask for the utmost highest white light of protection'.

Then, set your intention as to how you want to use it – as a protective shield, a healing or cleansing energy, etc.

Finally, imagine the white light surrounding, or being directed to, where you would like it to be.

Astral Plane

The Astral Plane
is a world of illusion
where everything
is produced
by thought.

There are no limitations or restrictions. You can travel anywhere, do anything, create whatever you desire. The limit to your creations and experiences are imposed upon you only by the limits of your imagination. Your thoughts manifest immediately into reality and your reality changes the instant your thoughts do.

And how does this happen?

Well, the astral plane is fluidic in nature because the vibrational rate of the energy is so much higher than your physical energy.

> *When you're operating under astral plane conditions, thoughts are moulded into form.*

Naturally, the reality is subjective, temporary and ever changing at this level of existence. It is your astral body, the fourth layer of the aura, which gets to visit this realm. You can access it while you sleep, during meditation, or by consciously willing yourself, and it's where your spirit goes between incarnations.

In general, the astral plane is often considered to be somewhere above you, which is a fairly logical assumption because the word 'astral' is related to the stars and we talk of 'higher' energies and floating upwards when we 'leave our bodies'.

> *But the astral plane is not literally 'up'. It exists all around you – left, right, front, back, up and down.*

You're not aware of it as you go about your day to day business because it's beyond your five physical senses. It has different 'floors', or levels, so to speak, and each floor resonates at a progressively higher rate and your energy can go to wherever it matches the resonance.

> ***Memories of the astral can be vague
> at best and non-existent at worst.***

But recollection ability aside, the astral plane has much to offer in the way of learning and during your astral travels you actively seek out teachers and guides who offer you assistance and anything else that will be conducive to your spiritual growth.

> *You receive a lot of guidance through your
> dreams so it's possible to pose a question
> to the Universe before going to sleep.*

Although you may not be able to recall your astral experience your energy will hold the answer to your question and you will access the information when you need it, usually via something like a brainstorm or moment of inspiration.

Apart from guides and teachers, the astral plane also houses other occupants. And it is these entities that usually get singled out for a mention so much more than any of the others. Residing in the lowest and densest realm of the astral, they are inclined to receive bad press because their energy leans more towards the negative than the positive and they are drawn to the 'dark' energies of an individual, such as fear, hate, depression, anger, etc. But each level of the astral deals with different types of reflections and there is always higher guidance on offer for these entities.

Naturally, it is the choice of these 'lower astral entities' to either stay put or raise their vibrations. Eventually each soul, when it is ready, will go on to its next stage of growth.

It pays to be aware of these entities because whenever you venture to the astral, asleep or otherwise, you take all your emotions with you so should you ever encounter a lower astral entity you have to accept you attracted their energy to you. Your vibration is being reflected back to you.

The astral plane shows you exactly what energy you are giving out because you only ever attract equal back.

In these revealing moments you have to take responsibility for what you are creating or drawing to yourself. The sending out of lower vibrational emotional energy is just going to see you take delivery of a pile more.

Meeting up with negative entities can seem scary but there are positives to come out of such experiences. Firstly, you are forced to acknowledge you are holding onto negative emotions. Once recognised, you can start working to overcome them. Secondly, you are given the opportunity to face your fears and defeat them.

The energy of the astral lends itself to constant change and manipulation by each and every individual's subjective thoughts so you have the power to consciously control the astral environment. By changing your thoughts and altering the charge of your energy, you can send an entity packing.

Facing your fears and doing something about them on the astral can then be translated to your physical environment.

Yin and Yang

The ancient Chinese philosophy that is Yin and Yang concerns itself with duality and balance.

The terms Yin and Yang are used to illustrate the point that every single thing within the system of the universe has an opposite and it is the dynamics caused by this relationship of opposites which allows all things to exist.

The forces of Yin and Yang are not hostile to one another, they are complementary. Neither are they separate from each other. They work together in unity.

It is appreciated that one cannot exist without the other and everything contains elements of both forces. This is exemplified by the Yin and Yang symbol - a circle with two tear-shaped figures, one black, one white, both of which contain a seed of its opposite. The circle represents all things; completeness.

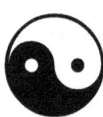

Some of the main principles of Yin and Yang are:

A thing can only exist in relationship to something else and whatever can be conceived of must have an opposite, otherwise it couldn't exist. 'Old' needs 'young' to define it, for example, because how else could 'old' exist as a concept?

Things 'divided' into Yin and Yang share essential qualities, which are categorised together because of their attributes – winter, cold, damp; summer, hot, dry. Because each thing gives way to the other and each thing is integral to the other, nothing is ever considered superior or inferior. Everything supports, nourishes and activates everything else.

A few of the assigned traits of Yin and Yang are:

Yin: feminine, moon, dark, night, low, contracting, soft, passive, cool, intuitive, emotional, anatomy, right brain, even numbers, Earth.

Yang: masculine, sun, light, day, high, expanding, hard, active, warm, logical, rational, physiology, left brain, odd numbers, Heaven.

*Because Yin is considered feminine
and Yang masculine this is not intended
to suggest anything about women and men in general.*

What Yin and Yang connote is not supposed to be literally applied to people as in, 'women equal this and men equal that'.

Yin and Yang are forces; observations of the construct of the universe.

Everything contains elements of both and if you can value this and embrace all the facets of yourself, you'll enjoy a balanced energy. Yin and Yang operate in mutual support of each other. If people hold the attitude that they are only one type of energy, imbalance is inevitable. The proof of this can be witnessed in society.

Duality can be found in the philosophies and religions of many cultures. We mention Yin and Yang not because it epitomises the forces of opposition, but because it tends to attract the most attention. But it doesn't matter what the concept is called, they all embody the basic laws of unity, harmony and balance.

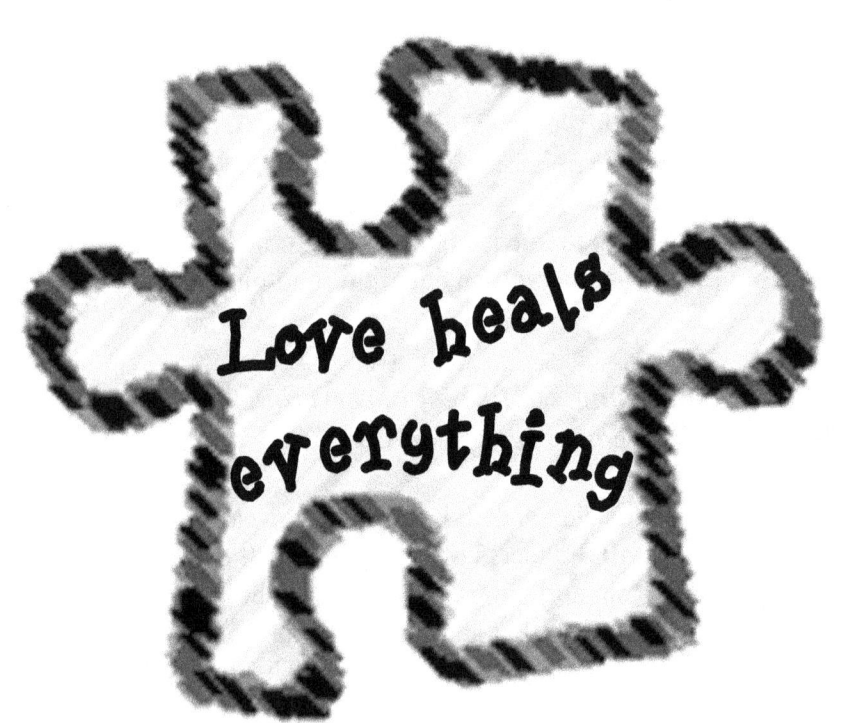

Ch'i and Meridians

Ch'i,
pronounced 'chee'
and also spelt Qi,
is a Chinese word which,
literally translated, means
air or breath.

Ch'i is vital, life force energy and, energy being energy, it makes up everything in the universe.

When the term ch'i is used in specific reference to the human body it is referring to the energy that is distributed throughout your body via your meridians.

Traditionally, the word meridian is used to denote the imaginary lines which circle the earth longitudinally from pole to pole. The lines are used to mark the different time zones around the globe. The meridians referred to here are also 'imaginary' in that they do not physically exist inside your body the way capillaries, veins and arteries do.

These channels, which are quite separate from those of your circulatory and nervous systems, are like electrical paths, or conduits, along which ch'i energy flows.

So, in reality, they do exist on an energy level and can be viewed or felt by a person who is sensitive to these energies.

Much of Chinese medicine is based around your meridians which can harbour sluggish energy or become blocked by holding onto unresolved emotional issues. Many of the healing techniques work on the principles of improving, enhancing and maintaining energy balance and flow so the body can enjoy strength, vitality and good health.

According to Traditional Chinese Medicine there are twelve channels of energy that flow through the body. They are grouped into the categories of YIN and YANG. Each Yin meridian has a corresponding Yang meridian and all are associated with emotions.

The Yin meridians are: heart, kidney, liver, lung, pericardium and spleen.

Yang: bladder, gall bladder, large intestine, small intestine, stomach and triple burner.

The pericardium is also sometimes referred to as circulation and the triple burner relates to heat production.

In addition to this there are also two central channels. They are the governor and conception meridians which regulate the other twelve and help to maintain the flow of energy within the entire system.

When the ch'i flowing through a meridian shows signs of stagnation or blockage it can be an indication that an aspect of that individual's emotional or mental state is out of balance in some way.

A knowledge of the emotional correlation of each meridian is a powerful tool which provides the healer with insight and understanding into the possible underlying reasons for the imbalance.

These include:

Bladder: anxiety, frustration, inner turmoil, willpower.
Gall bladder: indecision, bitterness, resentment, overwork, irritation, impatience.
Heart: love, forgiveness, compassion, empathy, lack of emotion.
Kidney: fear.
Liver: anger, rage, irritability, out of control.
Lung: holding onto grief and unresolved sadness; guilt.

Large intestine: usually an inability to 'let go'; too much 'holding on'. Hoarders.

Pericardium / circulation: regret, remorse, jealousy.

Small Intestine: resistance to change, oversensitive, fed up.

Spleen: feelings of self pity, insecurity, denial, envy, worry. Issues relating to a lack of self worth.

Stomach: hunger, greed, loneliness, nausea, disgust. Discontented, inadequate.

Triple Burner: despair, hopelessness.

Understanding and working with the meridians in this way makes this form of therapy a powerful healing modality.

Treatments such as acupuncture, acupressure and some forms of massage stimulate the energy flow along the meridians, unblocking, clearing and bringing balance and harmony back to all your systems. To assist healing, ch'i energy can also be placed into the body.

Apart from different healing techniques, a series of orchestrated movements known as Ch'i Gong (which is pronounced Kung and means 'work') also help to clear the meridians and restore normal health and normal energy flow.

As a point of interest, this same energy is referred to as 'prana' in India and as 'ki' in Japan.

Feng Shui

Pronounced
Fung Shway.

The art of Feng Shui,
which in Chinese means
'wind' and 'water',
is the study of the
hidden energy currents
and forces covering the
surface of the earth.

The 'wind' aspect represents the flow of the universal energy, or ch'i, which affects everything, while the 'water' represents the container or receiver of ch'i. Feng Shui principles are designed to harmonise the 'wind' and 'water' influences.

This ancient Chinese art and science teaches you to create a living and working environment that is balanced and harmonious; a place where you feel comfortable, happy and peaceful and somewhere you want to be.

Balancing the flow of energy through the placement of objects, furnishings and even knick-knacks to create happiness and harmony is its most basic principle.

Just as a balanced flow of ch'i within your body is conducive to your health, smooth, flowing energy in your environment is also imperative for your well-being. Enhancing the quality of the energy can improve your constitution, relationships, career, wealth. In fact, any areas of your life which you feel need improving.

Because Feng Shui is all about energy, your instincts, intuition and gut feelings about the best ways to create a harmonious environment shouldn't be dismissed. If it feels right - it is, but there are guidelines which can be implemented to help get you started.

Energetically, an area or room is divided into nine sections, each of which pertains to different aspects of your life.

This is known as the '**Bagua**'.

These areas are:

Wealth	Fame	Relationships
Family/ Health	Tai Chi ☯	Creative/ Children/ Projects
Inner Knowledge/ Intuition	Career	Helpful People/ Travel

If a specific area of your life felt as if it was stagnating you would use the Bagua to pinpoint the particular area within a room so you could set about reorganising things to recharge the energy and get it flowing smoothly again.

Let's say your relationship needed an overhaul. In the relationship corner of your home, or the appropriate area within any room of your home, you would need to have things that represent unity, togetherness and love. Ideally, then, you could place pairs of things such as photos of you and your partner, doves, hearts and other symbols of love.

Quotes, sayings and affirmations pertaining to love and marriage are nice and, if you are married, display honeymoon mementos, anniversary gifts and romantic holiday souvenirs. Further enhance the positive energy vibrations with the use of colour which, for relationships, is red, white and pink.

Candle Magic: Yellow for Confidence

Feng Shui is about location, location, location.

It is the correct placement of things which serves to slow down the gentle flow of ch'i without hindering it.

When ch'i flows slowly and smoothly your own energy picks up on it and matches its harmony.

Sense the ch'i in your environment and, the better it is, the better you will be because, just as good Feng Shui offers balance and harmony, living and working in an environment that doesn't feel right can have a detrimental effect on your well-being. So have fun, spruce up your areas, remove clutter and place objects and colours specific to your energy needs.

Additionally, the Chinese also advocate the advantages of a harmonious combination, arrangement and balance of the five elements of wood, fire, earth, metal and water. This can be done in a number of ways through the use of objects, shape and colour. In books that refer more to the Western style of Feng Shui, the focus for achieving harmony in your environment and personal space may be on the four primary elements of earth, air, fire and water.

What is talked about here hasn't even scratched the surface of this very involved subject. Many good books, going into greater detail, have been written about this wonderful art enabling you to open up a remarkable world of discovery.

***Feng Shui benefits everybody.
To spend time in a home or work place that feels right can be very uplifting, contributing to a more positive outlook on life.***

Death

Death is never easy
and it is a subject
most of us prefer not
to think or talk about.

It's an issue we tend to tip-toe around and speak about in whispers. People love to hear all the details of a birth but think it is morbid, even disrespectful, to discuss a death.

Why does the subject make so many people feel very uncomfortable? What are we so afraid of?

Do we believe that if we don't talk about it, it won't happen to us or we can pretend it hasn't happened to somebody else? Is it because the emotions associated with death are such painful ones?

To the very core of our being we feel such things as anguish, agony, grief, heartbreak, loss, injustice. Death grips our hearts and squeezes mercilessly.

If we suffer a deeply personal loss we often believe we will never recover – such is the intensity of our thoroughly overwhelming emotions.

Yes, we miss the physical presence of the deceased and we need to experience a period of grieving to help us release the emotions we're feeling, but understand -

no person ever leaves this planet without the soul having chosen to go.

This includes life whilst it is still forming, babies and children.

Death is the soul's way of letting us know its purpose in this life has been completed, whether a life was lived or not. The death of a baby, for instance, could indicate that its soul's purpose was to trigger a particular lesson for the parents. After all, we are both teacher and student.

Even the highly personal choice to voluntarily terminate a pregnancy is made by more than the expectant woman, or couple. Again, the spirit of the embryo or foetus has had input into the fate of all parties concerned with the decision. The emotional impact such a decision can have has the capacity to adversely affect the rest of a person's life. But every feeling felt, whether it be guilt, shame, fear, remorse, sadness, or even inconvenience, and every moment spent thinking about the termination or pondering the final choice is designed to be a lesson of some description.

And it's important to find the lesson, respect it and learn something from it so the same decision doesn't have to be made time and again.

Because the soul concerns itself with growth, it has no need to linger on and on when the time has come for it to move on so it simply 'slips away' to prepare for its next incarnation. Death of the physical body means rebirth of the soul into the world of spirit where it returns to its natural state and a new beginning.

Remember – we are spiritual beings having physical existences so DEATH could easily be an acronym for:

Departing Earth And Travelling Home.

Because we forget we are spirits first, for many people life in the physical body is the be all and end all. We identify with, and value, this aspect of ourselves so greatly that we are reluctant to let it go. Ironically though, we suddenly value it more at the time of impending death than ever before! And that goes not only for our own body, but other people's as well! When a loved one's time has come to pass over we cling desperately, we deny, we judge, we rage, we cry, we bargain, we clutch, we take control by telling them they aren't going anywhere. They are staying with us because that is what we want and surely that is what they must want also. They can't go – we need them, love them, can't live without them.

> ***But face the facts, the day will come when every single one of us will leave this planet.***

No one says that has to cancel out the way you feel about those you love but knowledge and education of the after death experience can do much to ease the uncertainty.

Much research on the subject of near-death experiences has been undertaken and written about by Dr. Elisabeth Kübler-Ross and makes for interesting reading. That extra bit of reassurance that such research provides can help to alleviate anxiety and bring more of a peaceful acceptance of the inevitable.

> *Connecting to your spiritual self, knowing your soul is eternal and having the faith to accept that you are not just your body, also helps.*

At the time of death your consciousness retracts its focus from the physical existence, much like it does when you're asleep and you become aware that other dimensions of reality exist. Some of these other dimensions you have experienced in your dream state.

Many great masters and metaphysical teachers tell us that as we create our reality on the earth plane, so too do we create our reality at the time of our death. In other words, when your spirit leaves your physical body you experience what you choose to, or what you expect to.

Your personal thoughts and beliefs about life after death will create for you that immediate experience. For example, if you hold a firm belief in the pearly gates of Heaven, you may witness that very thing. And they'll look just as you always believed they would. Perhaps you're expecting to see a mode of transportation that will whisk you away or you believe loved ones, relatives and pets who are deceased, even angels, will all be there to greet you. If you wish them to be, they will. Should you harbour strong fears of burning in the fires of hell with Lucifer jabbing at you with a searing pitchfork … well you may even create that too if you believe it enough.

Whichever scenario you find yourself in the middle of, even nothingness, lasts only a short period of time until the hallucination fades away and you become aware of the reality of the spirit world and remember who you really are.

All these states are temporary and there are those in spirit who are there to assist you with the transition from one plane of existence to another and sometimes your spirit needs a bit of extra help as it doesn't always float off to the spiritual realm in an organised and orderly fashion.

A spirit can become 'earthbound', that is, unable to leave the denser energies of the physical realm, for any number of reasons such as - after a sudden accident a person may be unaware they have actually died so the spirit might cling to the familiarity of the physical, or they may have a strong pull to people, places or possessions still on Earth and are reluctant to leave. However it happens, when a spirit is dazed and confused and can't find its way back to the higher realms, it's called a 'lost soul'.

Fortunately, there are 'lost soul' rescue teams.

There are those in spirit, or people 'out of their body' while they sleep, who perform the work of guiding these lost souls 'to the light', which essentially is a beacon. Some people who have had near death experiences talk of going towards a brilliant white light at the end of a tunnel, or something similar. And the light is there – as a guide to reaching the higher energies and to shine the way for a spirit's journey home.

Those who perform rescues remind the lost soul of their spiritual nature and explain the reality of what has happened to them.

They encourage them to leave the lower realm and move on to where they need to be so their spirit can get back on the growth and evolvement track. They then assist the spirit to the light.

Because we're human and we have human emotions, death can seem so cruel. People we love are 'snatched' away from us and it is sad that we don't always have the opportunity to say goodbye. But just because someone has left the physical doesn't mean communication with them has to cease. If you feel the need, you can speak to their spirit, write them a letter or connect with them in your dreams. You can do this yourself, if that is what your heart desires, so there is no real need to consult a medium or a psychic.

Know and trust that you are heard and understood by the person you need to express yourself to.

You are always connected by the energy bonds of strong emotional attachment and you can take comfort in the knowledge that you are never really apart, or alone.

Sometimes people pass over and you may feel that there were aspects to the relationship that needed healing; that there were unresolved hurts and issues. They hurt you. You hurt them. It doesn't really matter which way it goes.

Luckily it's never too late to heal and forgive.

Remember, they are only a thought away and you can send them love, healing, forgiveness, or apologies and they may very well be sending you the same things back. There are no obstacles to love and healing, only the illusions and barriers you create.

Imagine what a different energy and attitude humans could create if, in some way, we chose to celebrate death for the freedom, release and rebirth that it brings. Loved ones could gather around the bed of a person ready to pass over, sending them love and light. Angels and spirit guides could be called in to assist in the spirit's transition.

Candles, crystals, flowers, fragrant oils, music, prayers and singing could aid in the celebration and completion of their life on Earth and, among the sadness, everybody could find the joy in the knowledge that a spirit is going home.

After all that you might be wondering what the delicate subject of death has to do specifically with energy? In the end it comes down to the truth that we are all the one energy from the one source expressing itself in different ways.

Simply, unemotionally and rationally, death is merely a change of form; a transition from one phase of being, to another.

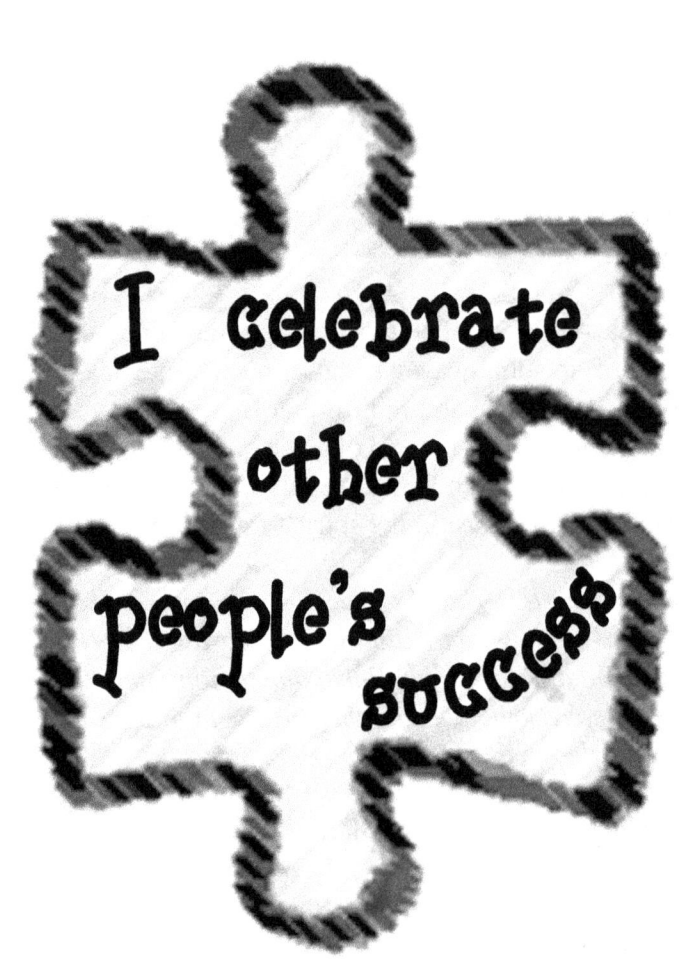

Reincarnation and Past Lives

Reincarnation
is the belief that
your spirit returns
time and time again,
to a new body, to live
many different lives.

You reincarnate by choice for the evolution of your spirit because, as we've already said, you desire to experience and create many different things that only your physical life can offer although some highly evolved beings incarnate out of service, to guide and teach you and to raise the consciousness of humanity.

When you die, your spirit 'leaves' your body and makes its way to the astral plane. Once there, you 'hang' around for awhile doing all manner of stuff. You might need to rest and heal if your death was traumatic.

You may choose to visit the halls of learning to expand on your knowledge to assist in your growth and evolution on the spiritual realm.

You may desire to offer guidance to those you are close to who are still living in the physical realm or you may choose to bask in the light and overwhelming love and peace that is the energy of your spirit.

Some spirits may stay in the astral realms and create for themselves a life similar to the one just experienced on Earth.

The soul always has free will and chooses to express its creative power any which way it desires.

When you're ready, with the help of spirit guides you review the life you have just led, decide what you did or didn't learn and then set about choosing what your next 'mission' will be.

Before you make your way back to the physical, you set your intentions and make certain choices; choices that will create for you environments, situations and relationships that are conducive to your growth and evolution.

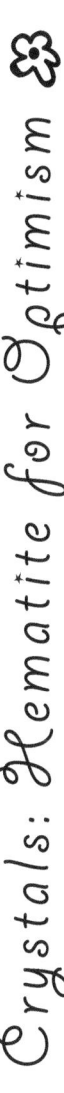

You choose your place and time of birth, your race, state of health, gender (you are not always exclusively male or female), and you even preselect your parents. Their souls have also chosen, at the spiritual level, to be a part of your life theme.

Once you're back in the physical realm you may not actively remember your choices and tasks but you are guided along the path you have set for yourself by those in spirit and your instincts are their messages and your soul memories.

But even the best laid plans can go astray because you have free will and you create your reality at all times with your thoughts, words and actions so there are many roads you will take in your attempts to arrive at your 'chosen' destination.

As frustrating as your life can get sometimes, free will is important for your growth.

If you never had to make a single decision or face a single dilemma because Spirit came and rescued you every time you strayed from your path, you just wouldn't be living your life. You are a creative being and this is all part of the creative process.

With the loving attitude of a parent that realises a child must 'do' in order to learn, Spirit knows you need to come to your own realisations, stand on your own two feet, overcome your fears, move forward of your own volition and actively go after what you desire.

But know that there are signs and lessons all around you designed to move you along to the next phase of your development. When you develop an awareness for what is happening in your life, you begin to recognise your patterns. If you acknowledge the issues you need to confront and work to resolve them, you learn and grow.

***<u>Past Lives</u>, naturally enough,
are all the lives you've lived prior to this one.***

When you reincarnate you bring memories with you, from your past lives, that you hold at a cellular and energetic level.

You possibly hold these memories for one, or several, reasons:

- you died before you had a chance to recognise or complete the lesson associated with them
- the knowledge contained within the energy may help you this lifetime
- an aspect of the life may have had a profound effect on you so you chose to experience something similar again
- karma.

These past life memories will manifest as experiences in this lifetime enabling you, if necessary, to process, resolve and clear this energy. This is especially true of karma. Also, many of your natural talents and abilities may be things you have worked at perfecting over many lives and by bringing the memory with you, you finally get to use your skills in the grandest way. Child prodigies would certainly fit that bill and Mozart is a fine example of that possibility.

Regression to past lives has been achieved through hypnotherapy and much of this work has been documented but if you're not quite sure about it all think about your own life for a moment and consider some of your choices and experiences.

Do you have an affinity for a particular culture?

Are you drawn to a certain style of jewellery, clothing, furnishings?

What period of history holds a fascination for you?

What biases and prejudices enrage you?

Have you ever had the sense that you 'knew' someone when you first met them?

Are there people you immediately clicked with?

Is there someone in your life you just can't get along with but have no discernible reason for why this is?

Most of the people you interact with, especially family, are all people you've known before and your relationship roles chop and change to suit your lessons.

You may have been married to your mother-in-law in a previous incarnation, for example. Yes, it's true!

Irrational fears and phobias may also be from past lives. If you have a fear of water yet have never had a bad experience to account for your reaction, you may have drowned in a previous incarnation. Don't like fire, cats, elevators, aeroplanes? If you really have no rational reason for your fears, your feelings of discomfort towards something could be from another time and place. You hold energy memories from all your lifetimes. Sometimes it takes you many tries to resolve an issue.

From our limited human perspective it is easy to judge other people's choices and behaviour but from a spiritual (bigger picture) point of view their experiences all have meaning and purpose and are no less, or more, important than your own. Each of us progresses at our own pace.

There are many themes and perspectives to experience and as many lifetimes as you need to experience them but the quicker you deal with your stuff, the quicker you contribute to your spirit's evolution and growth.

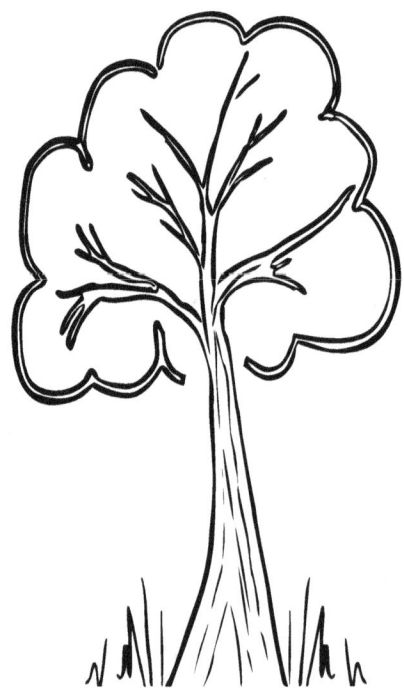

Karma

Karma is a term
derived from the
Sanskrit meaning 'deed'.

Fundamentally, the concept states that the results of your thoughts, words and actions will determine your state of life and also your destiny or fate in your next incarnation. It is the notion that you will always experience for yourself whatever it is you 'give out'. As the sayings go – 'What goes around comes around'; 'You reap what you sow'; 'You get back what you give out'.

Karma dictates laws of cause and effect so every action has its own consequences.

Being a natural universal law which follows that like attracts like, karma appears to both punish and reward. However, the energy of karma is neutral. It doesn't make an active decision about right or wrong, good or bad. These judgements are human, physical things.

The energy that comes back, quite simply, is the energy that got sent out.

Your outer world is a reflection of your inner world. It's feedback, like looking in a mirror. Karma teaches you to be mindful of the energy you do send out. If you pay attention to what is being returned, you get the chance to gain personal insights and increase your self-awareness.

Karma is also necessary so you can understand about balance; about the polarity of things. You need to experience both sides of something in order to understand it in a well-rounded way. For example, if you steal, chances are you will get stolen from.

Ultimately, karma occurs for the growth, evolvement and experience of your soul.

Colour

Colour surrounds us;
it is absolutely
everywhere.

It is generally accepted that certain colours can have particular effects on us and people have attached meaning to colour.

For example: red roses represent love and passion. We know about 'mood lighting' and we wear specific colours during certain rituals or ceremonies. Western society widely accepts black for funerals and white for weddings.

> *Many things around you influence you in so many ways every day, without you being aware of it, and colour has that same influence.*

Throughout your life you may change your colour preferences many times. The way you decorate your home is a good indication of how you are feeling at any given time. By that we mean that the colours you are attracted to could indicate your true inner state and measuring your choices against the colours of your chakras is usually a good indication of what sorts of things you might need to fill your life with, or what issues are relevant to you at that time.

> *For instance, being attracted to blue may mean you need to speak up more; orange might mean you're getting ready to start using your personal power.*

You can bring colour into your life in many different ways. There are flowers, lights, clothes, materials, scarves, food, paint, décor, candles, crystals and even visualising colour during meditation and breathing it into the body.

Colours also influence the way you look at people. Imagine if you were conducting business with a man. You had only ever spoken with him on the phone and, by his manner and speech, you had built a mental picture. What would happen if, when you finally met this man, he was wearing a lavender, pink, or powder blue suit instead of a more traditional dark colour?

You might make a judgement about him, possibly an unfavourable one, because he didn't look or present how you 'expected'. You might discount the positive image you had previously built and turn it into a negative one. You would probably do this unconsciously. This goes to show the important role colour plays. What colours he is wearing shouldn't make a difference, but somehow they do.

By utilising the power contained within a colour to evoke certain psychological, physical, emotional and spiritual responses colours can heal too, bringing relief to ailments and helping you balance your energies.

Through their experiences, colour practitioners have found that specific colours are beneficial for helping eliminate all manner of ailments.

Energy vibrations of particular colours used in décor also enhance the properties of rooms in the home.

Red is helpful for varicose veins, anaemia, coldness and tiredness. Because red is an energising colour it is ideal for activity areas and passages. Not recommended for a child's bedroom, offices, factories, or stress areas.

Orange is suitable to help with the common cold, constipation and depression. The uplifting properties of orange make it a wonderful colour to have in entertainment and dining areas. Not recommended for bedrooms or study areas.

Yellow is beneficial for hepatitis, jaundice and rheumatism. Yellow décor is best used in rooms where solitary activities are undertaken, like a study room, because of its focus and mental activity properties. Not recommended for use in bedrooms.

Green helps with painful joints, migraines, sprains and strains, chest pains, heart disease, tumours and warts. Green décor is great in healing areas or convalescing rooms. Not really for use in living or activity areas.

Blue benefits arthritic joints, asthma, anxiety, burns, coughs, fever and itching. Wrapping a blue scarf around a sore throat helps to ease the pain. If you're having trouble sleeping or relaxing, blue is a great colour to paint your bedroom. A wonderful colour to use in a healing or treatment room. Not recommended for use in dining rooms or entertainment areas.

Turquoise is used for cases of asthma, catarrh, cold sores, hay fever and stings. This greenish-blue colour is lovely for bathrooms and kitchens. Not for activity or play areas.

Violet helps with conjunctivitis and mental illness. The spiritual aspects of violet make the hue ideal for places of prayer and meditation. Not really suitable for use in wards or treatment rooms.

Magenta can alleviate fainting, headaches and morning sickness and is recommended for use in entrance halls, chapels and lecture rooms. Not for entertainment rooms.

Remember, always go with what you instinctively feel. Colour choice is still a very personal thing. You don't have to decorate your home garishly but placing an item of the appropriate colour in the specified rooms can't do any harm. Experiment and go with your own feelings.

As babies, from the moment we can focus our eyes, bright colours attract and hold our attention.

Colour enlivens our spirit and helps us express many things we sometimes cannot adequately put into words. Colours give a wealth of information and they are important for our general well-being. Who doesn't feel a sense of delight at seeing a rainbow?

Can you imagine what the world would be like if all we saw was black, white and grey and how that kind of dreary drabness would affect moods?

Colours heal and colours evoke emotions. Appreciate and enjoy them. Use them to support you and bring out the best, most positive qualities you possess.

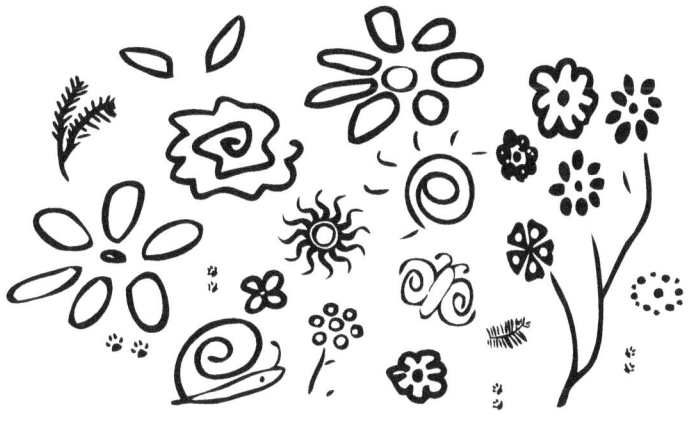

Oils: Frankincense for Courage

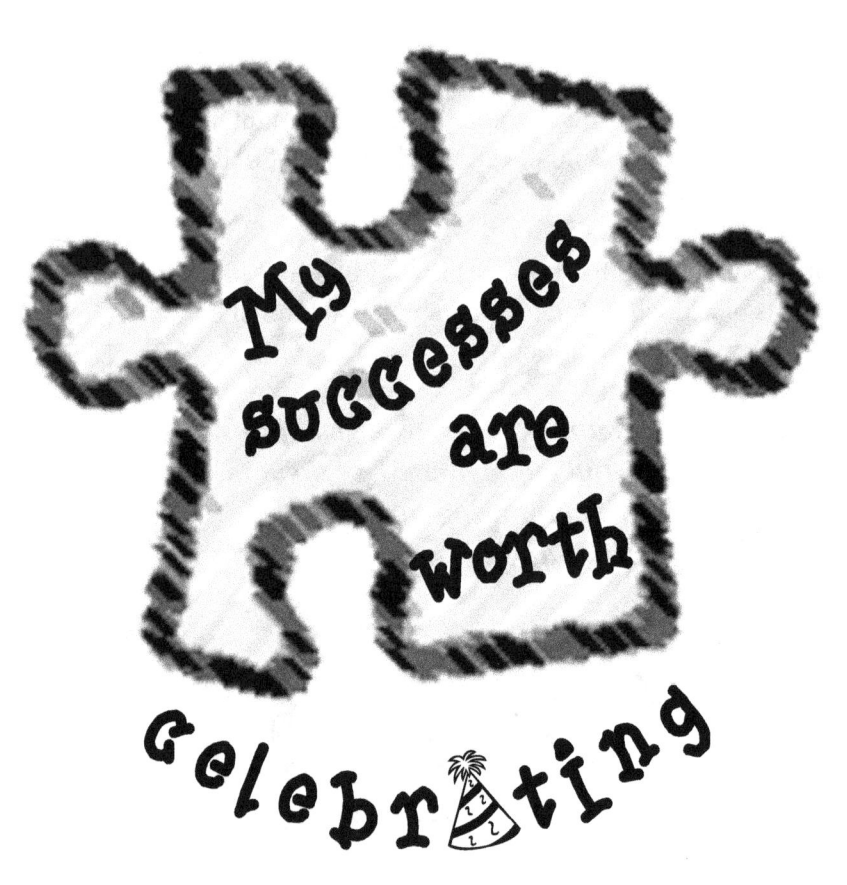

Psychic Phenomena

The word 'psychic' means: forces or mental processes outside the possibilities defined by natural or scientific laws.

Phenomena describes remarkable and extraordinary occurrences or people.

In other words – psychic phenomena are things that defy explanation because, more often than not, they're things that can't be measured by us in a seen-it-with-our-own-eyes, got-absolute-proof, kind of way.

*What we can't explain we're usually
wary of, and even suspicious.*

We're just not sure what to believe and we need substantial evidence to back up claims. But, as with the third eye, we're willing to give psychic stuff some credence because we're not totally disconnected from our spirits.

People are also referred to as being psychic. A psychic is someone who possesses highly developed intuitive skills.

There are many different categories of phenomena which fall under the umbrella of psychic happenings. Some of these include:

CARTOMANCY: Is the term used to describe divination using cards. The most popular and common cards used are the tarot. The illustrated cards, of which there are seventy-eight in a traditional deck, can be laid out in many different configurations and each card can be read alone and then jointly with those around it. There are many interpretations for the cards, because each reading is so intensely personal, so it is important that the reader always go with what they feel and not just rely on the suggested meanings of each card.

CHANNELLING: Channelling is the act of receiving information from the higher realms. Channels are like radios – receptacles that pick up on the invisible, yet real, sound waves all around us. To some degree you are a channel, even though you may not be aware of it. You channel assistance and guidance when you need it. You bring energy, information and light from the higher realms into the physical to enrich your life, aid in your development and give yourself a greater understanding of the non-physical realms. Channelling keeps your connection to the spirit realm alive and it gives you a higher level of information because you are working above your ego. Channelling, unlike Trance Channelling, is not an altered state.

TRANCE CHANNELLING: Through entering into an altered state of consciousness, or a trance, an individual becomes the physical means through which a spirit is able to communicate information. The spirit speaks directly through the person.

CLAIRAUDIENCE: means – 'clear hearing'. It is the ability to hear voices and sounds which are not audible to normal hearing. The voices can come from spirit guides. Clairaudients are usually able to discern between their own inner dialogue and the 'higher' voice of guidance.

CLAIRSENTIENCE: means – 'clear sensing'. It is the ability to 'feel' information rather than audibly hear it, or visually see it. A clairsentient might say something like: 'I feel you are not happy with your job'. They pick up on the energies which are affecting you emotionally and physically. This superphysical sense can also include smell, taste and touch.

CLAIRVOYANCE: means – 'clear seeing'. It is the ability to sense things which fall outside the range of your physical senses, usually via the 'seeing' of images or pictures. Clairvoyants use this 'sixth sense' to gain all manner of information like past, present and probable future events. Normally, some form of communication with spirit entities is required.

DOWSING: With the use of tools such as forked sticks, bent wire and pendulums, the ancient art of dowsing, as a means of divination, is used to locate people, objects and substances such as water. When the thing in question is located, the dowsing tool responds via spontaneous movement. Amongst other uses, pendulums can also be used to seek answers to 'yes' and 'no' questions. The pendulum moves in a circular fashion or swings in a straight line to indicate its response.

EXTRASENSORY PERCEPTION (ESP): Is the term used to describe the ability to perceive things that are not comprehensible within the realms of normal sensory activity. It is also called 'second sight'. To illustrate the true scope of perception that ESP encompasses, psychokinetic, telepathic, clairvoyant, clairsentient and clairaudient abilities make up its definition.

I CHING: ('ee cheeng') Also known as 'The Book of Changes', is an ancient Chinese oracle which gives the user an insight into the forces, literally 'the changes', that are occurring at any particular moment in time. The book was originally written to keep people in touch with the flow of universal life energy and information buried in the unconscious. The I Ching consists of a set of sixty four hexagrams (six lined figures.) Each hexagram, which has a name and a set of words or phrases that describe it, is made up of a combination of solid and broken lines. When a person chooses to consult the I Ching, a question is concentrated upon and an answer is sought by using yarrow sticks or casting three identical coins a total of six times. Each toss of the coins reveals a line of the hexagram.

When the six line hexagram is complete, its meaning can be interpreted. Insight is gained into the hidden energies and tendencies underlying the situation in question.

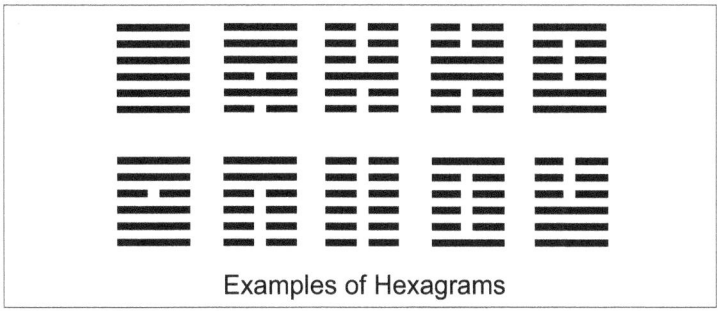

Examples of Hexagrams

NUMEROLOGY: Is a system based on numbers which are ascribed a mystical and magical meaning to ascertain a person's personality, destiny and life path. Usually dates of birth and names which have been converted from letters into their corresponding numerals, are added up. Should the figure be greater than nine it is systematically reduced to a single digit by adding each digit together. For example: if your total sum was 33 you would add 3+3 to get the symbolic number 6.

OUT-OF-BODY EXPERIENCE (OBE): Also called '**astral projection**' or '**astral travel**'. It is the experience of one's astral body, which is the fourth layer of the aura, separating itself from the physical body and travelling to the astral plane. It is believed that the astral body is attached to the physical body by a 'silver cord'. This connection is necessary to enable it to return. Some people are able to have an OBE at will and many people can dictate where they'd like to go and then recall the experience afterwards. It is commonly held that everyone astral travels whilst they're asleep, usually retaining very little memory of the occurrence when they awaken. It is suggested that any dreams you have where you are flying are usually remembrances of your astral travels.

PALMISTRY: A means of divination whereby the lines, mounds, fingers, thumbs and nails of the hands are 'read'. Most information is obtained from the lines on the palms which are said to reveal character and destiny. Each line, finger, mound and whorl has its own distinct meaning. Factors such as health, intellect, life expectancy, money, fate, career and love are indicated. Sizes and shapes of the hands and fingers are as important as the lines themselves. Even where a person chooses to wear their rings is considered important.

PSYCHOKINESIS (PK): Is the ability to alter the state of an object without using any physical force. It is considered to be achieved by using mind over matter. Objects can be bent or misshapen just by 'willing' them to be.

PSYCHOMETRY: Is the ability to sense or read energies from personal objects such as jewellery or keys. A reading is usually taken from an item the person frequently carries with them. Objects are imbued with all manner of energies and retain vibrations from the past. During the reading, the object is constantly held in the reader's hand and information is imparted according to what is sensed.

RUNES: The word 'runes' refers to an alphabetic script used by the ancient Germanic and Norse peoples. The script, or runic symbols, took on sacred meanings and although most of the wisdom of the ancient Rune Masters was taken with them to the grave, much work has since been done in the area of accurate and appropriate interpretation. It is said that so ancient are the runes their appearance qualifies them as the oldest, truly western oracle we possess. (The word 'oracle' refers to a medium through which Divine communication arrives.) The symbolic markings, or glyphs, have been carved or burnt into pieces of hardwood, incised on metal, or cut into leather and the runes can be consulted for support, guidance and self counselling. They are a tool for assisting you to guide your life in the present and a means of putting you in touch with your higher self to keep you on track. No special skills or abilities are needed to consult the runes.

👁 In your mind, clearly focus on an issue. Ask a question, draw a rune and refer to a book of rune interpretations. It's that easy. There are many different spreads that can give a greater overview of a situation. Anyone can make a set of runes using the likes of short sticks, bones, crystals, clay or, flat pebbles.

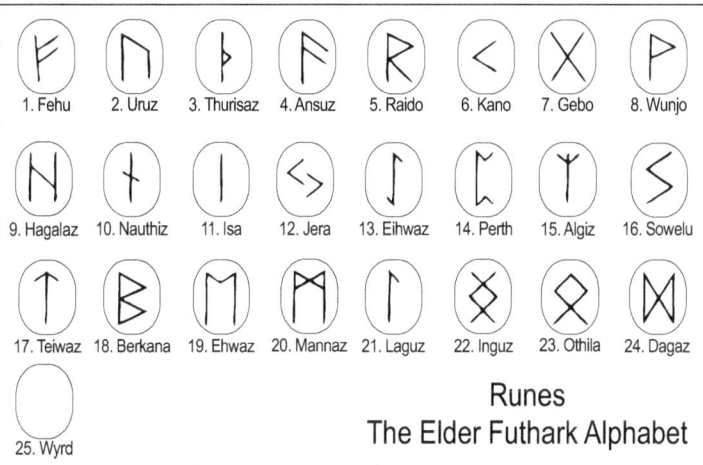

Runes
The Elder Futhark Alphabet

SCRYING: Is the name used for the method of divination which entails gazing into crystal balls, shiny stones, mirrors, or other reflective surfaces until visions and answers to questions are revealed.

TELEKINESIS: Is the power to move something by simply thinking about it and not using any physical force. Stationary objects can be made to move or float and items can be overturned.

TELEPATHY: Also known as **'mind reading'** or **'thought transference'**. Telepathy communicates thoughts, images and sensations from one person to another. Keeping within the natural laws of the universe, it is considered invasive to read someone else's thoughts without their permission and an infringement upon their privacy.

What most of the above phenomena really boils down to is the ability of the psychics to tune into the energies around them.

Some psychics use 'tools' such as cards, jewellery and crystal balls to help with their divination. Many others don't. Often times, the tool being used by the psychic is there to help focus the psychic energy so allowing the vision or information to be expressed in a clear and accurate manner. Each person feels comfortable working with different things in different ways.

An important point to be aware of is that being psychic doesn't necessarily mean being spiritual. They are two distinct things.

Psychic people aren't always spiritual and spiritual people aren't always psychic.

PSYCHIC VS SPIRITUAL: There are no rules that say a person who has developed their ability to tune into the energies around them also has to be a person who embraces spiritual principles. If ever you choose to consult a psychic for guidance, support, or help it is always a good idea to use your intuition and discernment to help you decide if the person's energy feels agreeable to your own and if you believe they will be able to meet your specific needs.

Trust your instincts because in any profession there are the 'good' and the 'bad' but know that there are genuine, loving souls out there waiting to assist you in your healing, whilst offering guidance for your personal and spiritual growth.

Here are some ways in which you might recognise a psychic who has your best interests at heart.

A spiritual psychic:
- Should not charge unusually high fees nor make outlandish claims or perform cheap parlour tricks.
- Will not claim to be an all-knowing guru, or an authority, or special, or 'chosen'.
- Is not competitive or puts other psychics down.
- Will not share personal information with anybody regarding other clients.
- Will not invade another's thoughts or space.
- Will not attempt to affect or influence the choices of another in any way.
- Will not impose their will on to others, or attempt to control the lives of others because a spiritual person knows you do not interfere with another's free will.
- Does not encourage clients to depend or rely on them.
- Is interested in empowering people to make their own decisions.
- Offers guidance and personal development counselling so that others can accept the responsibility for making their own life decisions.
- Possibly assists the client to become aware of the blocks that are preventing them from moving forward and having what they really want out of life.
- Assists the client in achieving clarity about the aspects of themselves and their lives that need healing.
- Quietly goes about their business not feeling they have to prove anything.

Live and let live

- Always uses discretion and tact.
- Will honour that ONLY YOU KNOW WHAT IS RIGHT FOR YOU.
- Will not expect you to accept anything as true unless it feels right for you.
- Will offer you information without passing judgement on your situation or feelings.
- Wants you to become self-reliant and self-assertive, to think for yourself and question what you are being told.
- Encourages you to develop your own psychic abilities and to know that all the answers are within you.
- Encourages you to trust in yourself and to act on your gut instincts, your deeper feelings and what your heart is telling you.

Ask yourself:
- Is their purpose and intention to genuinely help and support me?
- Are they a channel for love and light?

The more you become aware of the power you possess and acknowledge the extent of your creative abilities, the less you will look outside yourself for guidance.

But until that time you want to know that if you seek the advice of a psychic, that person will have your highest good at heart.

You are on a very personal and individual journey so a true spiritual teacher, whose purpose is to serve, will guide you and then step aside.

They know you hold the key to developing and knowing your personal self.

Spirit Entities/Guides/ Angels/Nature Spirits

By definition, these four forms of energy are quite distinct from one another.

SPIRIT ENTITIES: Apparitions, ghosts, phantoms, presences, spectres, spirits. These are some of the words which best describe spirit entities. Oftentimes they are the spirits of the deceased and the entities can be either human or animal. Spirit entities could probably be classified as 'general' spirits in that they don't necessarily confine themselves to one place or specific people and their purposes aren't necessarily fixed either.

Spirit entities are all around you and sometimes they make their presence known.

They do this in various ways, such as moving objects from place to place or manifesting strange smells. Some entities may appear in solid, material form whilst others appear transparent or even luminous.

If an entity lets their presence be known, it is usually for a specific reason such as delivering a message of some sort or comforting a grieving relative.

Other good indicators that an entity is near are hard to explain noises and voices, all over body shivers when it's not cold, strange sensations on the skin, a sudden awareness of heat or the uncanny sense of a lingering presence.

SPIRIT GUIDES: Unlike the spirit entities, spirit guides generally have defined purposes. Their role is like that of a teacher and they are there to guide you and keep you on track in respects to your life purpose.

A particular guide may stay with you over hundreds of lifetimes and be there to assist you when you leave the physical and return to spirit.

Here in the physical they can project energy to you, usually via thoughts and ideas. The guidance and information they offer you in this way can best be described as a sudden burst of inspiration or the unexpected solution to a problem which was previously elusive.

Spirit guides are many and varied and they usually have an area of expertise.

There are guides for creativity, employment, money, healing and luck, just to name a few. You can call upon any of the spirit guides, at any time, to assist you with any area of your life. Their help is always at hand. All you need to do is ask for it.

ANGELS: The word 'Angel', which means 'Messenger', is a derivative of both the Greek 'angelos' and the Roman 'angelus'

Angels act as intermediaries between the higher spiritual realms and humankind and they don't need to be associated exclusively with religion.

They have a hierarchical structure and there are nine orders of angels. In descending order they are:

seraphim, cherubim, thrones, dominations/dominions, virtues, powers, principalities, archangels and angels.

Each order have their own special purposes and tasks.

Angels work with your soul to remind you there is goodness and beauty in all things. When we think of angels, some of the words we associate are love, tenderness, beauty and nurturing. Energetically, they exist on a different vibrational level. Those who are tuned into that level are able to see them. Those of us who may not be able to perceive them fully with our physical senses can often still feel their energetic presence or feel them working in our lives.

If you feel such a connection or affinity for these gentle creatures, trust your inner senses and accept that they are sharing your life.

Even if some of us can't feel or see them it shouldn't stop us from believing they are there. We all have guardian angels who watch over, protect and guide us.

When it comes to unconditional beliefs, many of us could take a few lessons from children. A lot of children accept angels without question because they are able to open out their energies and connect to the energies of their angels. This is because children do not restrict themselves to science; that is until they get ridiculed for believing in something that 'isn't real' just because it can't be seen. Where is the harm for children, or adults, to take comfort in the knowledge that angels are watching over them; providing them with assistance, protection and guidance?

Angels are always with you and they work with you for your highest good. See them for what they are - beings of light who are filled with love and kindness for each and every one of us.

NATURE SPIRITS: Just as you have a spirit, so too does *every* aspect of nature - rocks, caves, trees, grass, flowers, water, crystals, *everything*. Nature spirits are many and varied and as diverse as nature itself but we know some of them as Elves, Fairies, Imps and Sprites. The four elements of nature also have spirits. We know these Elemental Beings as: **Salamanders** (Fire), **Gnomes** (Earth), **Sylphs** (Air), and **Undines** (Water).

Energetically, nature spirits vibrate at a different rate and work in different dimensions so we can't always have the 'solid' proof we'd like that they are everywhere, but the simple rule is: physical aspect = spiritual aspect. Just notice how you feel when you are surrounded by nature. Allow yourself to receive the feelings of abundance, joy and peace the nature spirits send out. Embracing this kind of positive energy is a wonderful thing.

As varied as they are in size, shape and disposition, many nature spirits possess a similar attribute in that they need human support to live and evolve because our surrounds are their homes. This factor is becoming a problem for them. The way in which we abuse nature is becoming dangerous for us and our nature spirit friends.

Each time we cut down a tree we are destroying a home. Each time we dig huge holes in the ground and rip out ores and minerals, we are destroying homes.

Humankind's lack of respect is disrupting nature in more ways than we are aware. We talk about the hole in the ozone layer and the ice caps melting but we speak only in terms of how these things affect our lives. The more things we rip out of the ground and the more things we destroy without compunction, the more nature will abandon us. And when the nature spirits leave our environment, our surrounds, which we take for granted, will no longer thrive because they now lack an energy they need.

Nature is alive and, like us, it needs its spirits to survive.

Oils: Lavender for Peace

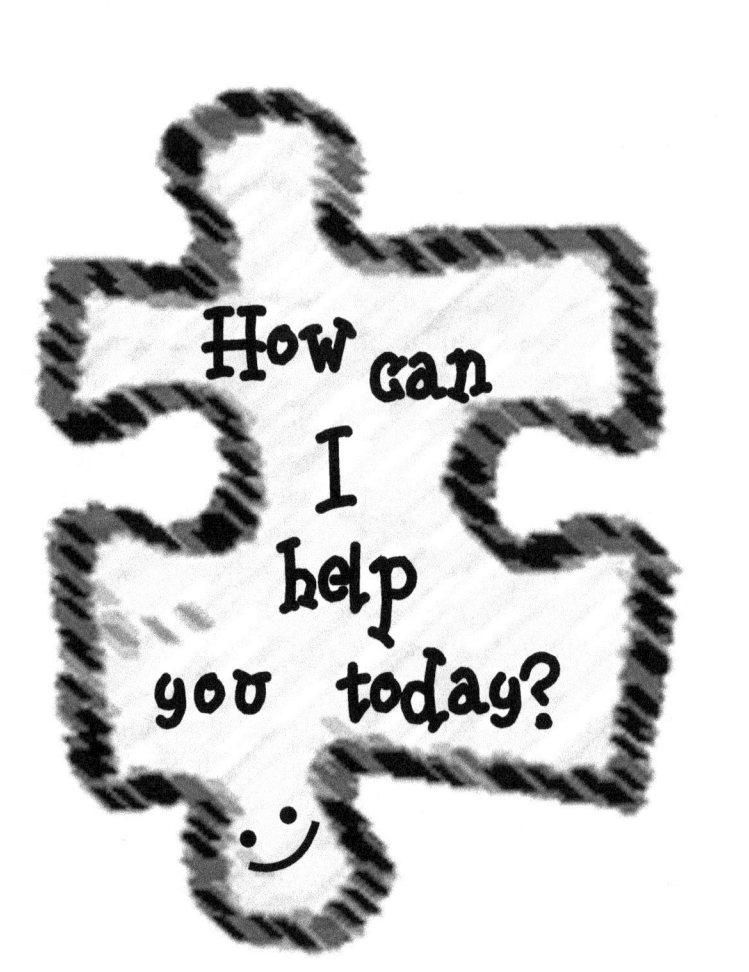

Meditation

Meditation is about stillness and silence; relaxation for the mind and body.

Meditation is deeply nurturing and deeply satisfying. It has much to offer and its benefits include:

- balancing of the mind, body and emotions
- deep relaxation and calmness
- a sense of inner peace and harmony
- healing on all levels of your being
- better sleep
- increased tolerance, positiveness and coping abilities
- health benefits associated with a de-stressed body, e.g. lower blood pressure
- connection with your spirit
- deeper insights into the self
- expanded spiritual awareness.

You're worthy of all this so give yourself the gift of some *you* time. Set aside twenty to thirty minutes a day to do it.

There are no absolute right or wrong ways to meditate. Do what feels right.

Generally, it is best to sit or lie comfortably. Soft music can help to focus the mind and quiet any incessant chatter about what you should be doing instead of meditating.

Relax and breathe, that's all you have to do.

Focus on your breath, in and out. Silently repeat a mantra such as 'Om' to help keep you in the moment.

Enjoy and appreciate being in the moment. Not yesterday. Not tomorrow. Now. Allow yourself the luxury of just being. Enjoy the time you are taking for yourself. Enjoy the peace. Enjoy the stillness. Enjoy the power of silence.

Also, progressive relaxation from toes to crown is an enjoyable way to meet your body and really get to know it.

Focus in on your heart centre; encourage self-love; breathe in positive energy and feel yourself radiating loving energy.

Fill your aura with healing colours. When you exhale, consciously blow out toxins. Feel them being expelled from every cell.

During this state of detached observation, be aware of any thoughts that pop in from your subconscious. Listen to what your inner self is telling you. The words may hold the solution to a problem.

Meditation helps you to integrate yourself with the spiritual dimension. This, in turn, helps to loosen the hold the physical world tends to have. The things you stress about in your life aren't so dire in the spiritual realm.

To make this valuable tool a part of your every day may take some discipline. Here are some suggestions:

- keep it simple
- practise it regularly
- attend meditation classes
- find a teacher or a group that meets on a regular basis
- read books on the subject
- use meditation tapes/CDs
- create a comfortable special place where you can take time for yourself to enter and connect with your inner world
- do it surrounded by nature.

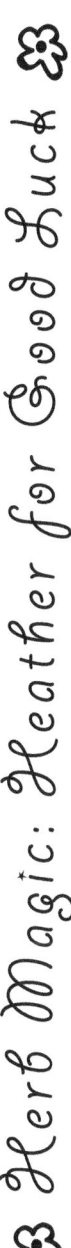

ॐ

The Spiritual Stuff Wrap Up

Spirit is a world of its own, with its own language and the concepts and definitions offered here have provided you with a broad base of knowledge about the world beyond this world.

Seeking out Spirit is exciting and including Spirit in your life becomes normal and part of your everyday.

Each of us is on our own personal journey with our own life lessons to learn. We are all at different stages of growth and evolvement. What you learnt in your last life others may be learning this life and vice versa.

What is true for you is right for you - even if it may not be right for someone else.

Each to their own. That's Spirit's way.

Always:
Trust your intuition.
Acknowledge your instinctive feelings.
Listen to your inner voice.

For these things are also the language of Spirit.

We are all connected.

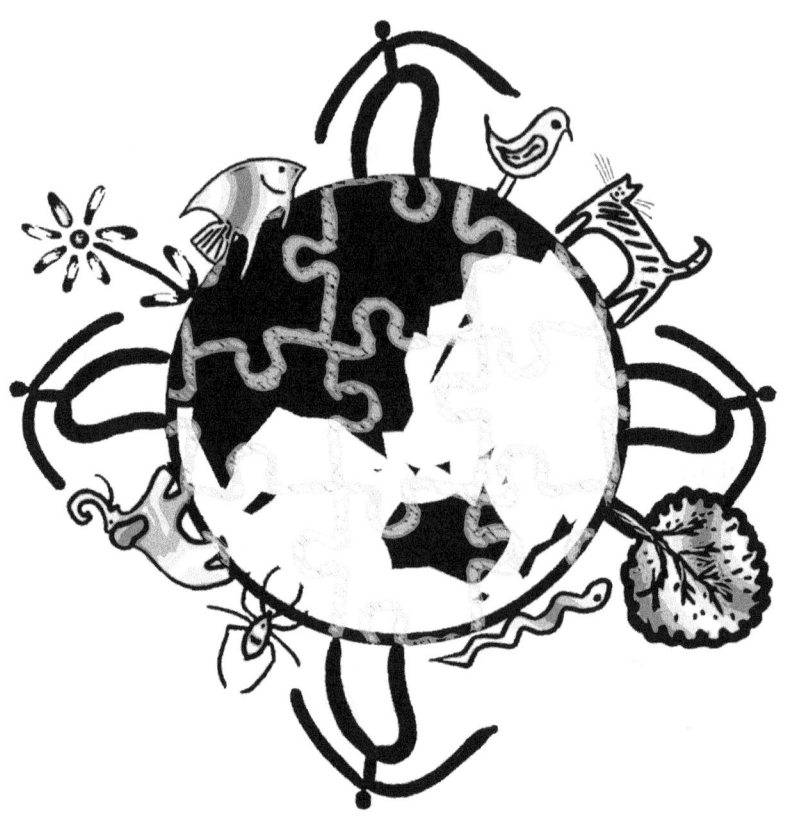

When we work together, all things are possible.

Body Symbolism

At the core of
every illness, injury
or addiction is an
emotional issue
waiting to be released.

We'll say that again:

At the core of every illness, injury or addiction is an emotional issue waiting to be released.

Your body tells you everything you need to know about your emotional state.

Often, though, the message is missed.

First, let's think about the obvious messages your body sends you – hunger means you need to eat; tiredness tells you to rest; shivering tells you to put on warm clothing. You accept these messages and act on them accordingly in the best interests of your comfort and health.

But what about cuts, bumps, bruises and burns? Could broken bones, disease, 'accidents' and even a cough have deeper meaning?

Absolutely.

Any illness or injury is a communication from your subconscious mind to your conscious mind. It's saying –

"Now I've got your attention via this ailment, let's figure out what the emotional issue is so it can be dealt with."

When the body manifests physically what you are suppressing emotionally, it's important to consider which part of the body is being affected as this helps to hone in on the issue.

This is known as 'body symbolism'.

Energetically, each part of your body means something.

Let's take a few examples.

What do you do with your arms? Arms carry things, they reach out and take for yourself what you need, they hold people close, or push them away.

Your legs move you along in life. They give you the ability to walk forward, or backward, and represent your direction.

Your spine and back are your support structure. Your shoulders bear a lot of responsibilities or burdens.

All your body systems are included in this - immune, reproductive, endocrine, etc. Joints, ligaments, blood, muscles, senses, and on and on.

Every cell. Every mass.

Now that you're thinking a bit deeper about your body, you can start asking questions about your ailments.

For example: if you have a cold, that means your immune system has been compromised and so your body's defences are down. Ask – 'Do I feel defenceless?' 'Am I able to fight for myself?' 'Where am I being attacked?'

If you have aches and pains in any of your joints, ask yourself about your ability to be flexible. Are you too rigid? Do you bend enough?

Suppressed emotions calling out to be released show up in the body in pretty much any ailment you can think of.

As an initial guide, the following may help you.

Are you experiencing problems with:

Blood: Represents joy; relating to family.

Chest: Is it congested? Are you feeling trapped or smothered; suffocated by others?

Cancer: One of the causes of cancer is considered to be the holding in of lots of bitterness, resentment and deep hurt. The emotions literally, physically eat away at the body. To further refine the issue, consider where in the body the cancer is.

Diabetes: Does life or love contain any sweetness or joy? Are you sabotaging your own happiness? Why?

Eyes or Ears: Is there something you don't want to see or hear?

Gall Bladder: Deals with bitterness and resentment. The word 'gall', in the non-medical sense, means impudence, irritation, anger, vexation, malevolence. This is a co-incidence.

Heart: Deals with the ability to give and receive love.

Kidneys: Represent fear. What are you afraid of?

Large Intestine: Represents the ability to 'let go'.

Liver: Represents anger. How much anger are you harbouring?

Lungs: Represent grief or guilt. How much of either are you holding onto?

Pancreas: Represents the sweetness and fullness of life. Are you getting the most out of your life? Are you benefitting?

Reproductive Organs: Represent how you view yourself as a man/woman. Also deals with sexual relationships. Is yours comfortable and happy? Or not?

Skin: Lets you know about your self image and self worth and how you feel you present yourself to the world.

Stomach: Represents the ability to process and assimilate ideas and experiences.

Throat: The communication centre. Are you able to speak your truth or be heard? If not - who is not allowing you to speak? Is your throat sore? Anger may be held there, unable to be expressed.

Body symbolism also looks at whether the manifestation of the ailment is on the left or right side of the body.

Narrowing the parameters in this way can help you zoom in on the probable emotional cause more quickly.

As in Yin and Yang, left represents feminine, the past and spiritual. If you manifest an illness, pain or injury on the left side of your body you can ask yourself questions in relation to these three aspects, which may provide greater insight and clarity.

For example, if you focus on the feminine aspect perhaps there are issues pertaining to a female in your life – mother, daughter, wife, sister, etc. Could it be that unresolved past events are triggering the current ailment or perhaps you've deviated too far from your spiritual purpose – growth, learning, chosen lessons?

The right side represents masculine, present time and the physical. Ask your body whether this is to do with a male, a situation happening now or, are your physical needs being met – work, rest, play?

In addition to the above, the things you purposely inflict upon yourself in the form of addictions are especially telling about your suppressed emotions.

Even though the whole body is ultimately affected by an addiction, initially a particular aspect of the self is specifically targeted. Here are some things to consider to help you get to the heart of any addictions and release them.

Food: The organ immediately affected is the stomach. Food addicts are trying to stave off feelings of emptiness; trying to fill a void. Compulsive eating is also a mask for nervousness and being scared.

Alcohol: Directly affects the liver. People who drink to excess are full of unexpressed anger.

Cigarettes: Smoke is taken deep into the lungs. Smokers are full of unexpressed grief.

Painkillers: Affect the kidneys. Addicts are full of fear.

Drugs: Such as heroin – are often administered directly into the blood stream. Drug addicts are full of deep sadness and pain. The first place to look for the cause would be around family. All addictions are a form of self-punishment but this one is particularly extreme.

Sugar: Addicts are trying to sweeten up their life. Sugar masks feelings of bitterness and resentment.

Caffeine: Is a stimulant. Addicts are masking feelings of despondency and boredom.

Gambling: The emotional issues associated with a gambling addiction are security and worth. An addict is trying to avoid feelings of insecurity and worthlessness.

Other addictions include things like: drama, fashion, cosmetic surgery, shopping, other people's lives. Addictions such as these, like all addictions, offer a form of escapism. They're something to fixate on so the real issues can be avoided for one more day.

*When the emotional issue is released
there is nothing there to hold the addiction
in place, so it just falls away.*

A good way to really get an understanding for body symbolism is to refer to a book on the subject such as Annette Noontil's, '*The Body Is The Barometer Of The Soul*' or '*You Can Heal Your Life*' by Louise L. Hay. The concepts discussed in these excellent books provide many insights.

Books on Shiatsu and Chinese medicine are also useful as they give reasons for imbalances along the energy meridians and in the associated body organs.

Also check the body part/chakra correlation.

Body symbolism is such an extensive topic and one well worth looking into, but you don't need to study it in any great depth to discover what your own illnesses/addictions mean.

Move your awareness to any area 'calling' for your attention and ask your body what it's holding there. Ask, 'What is the emotional representation of the pain, illness or addiction?' Notice the first thoughts, feelings, or memories that come to you. Trust your instincts.

By taking the time to connect to your physical body; to listen, tune in and pay attention to it, you can decipher the meaning of its communication.

Body symbolism is also an excellent tool for helping you to determine any emotional issues that are affecting your children.

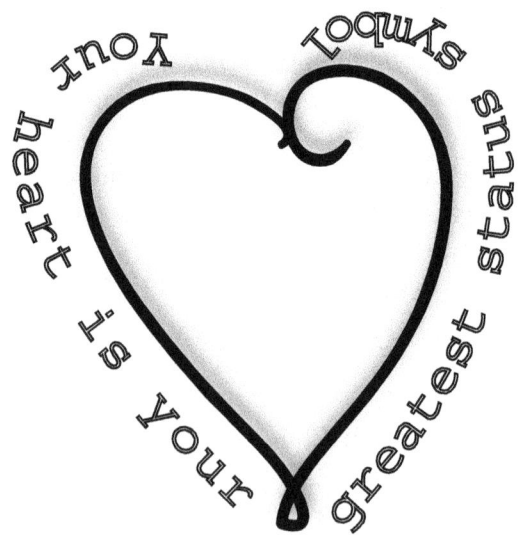

Your heart is your greatest status symbol

Alternative Healing

Alternative Healing is the oft used expression which aims to set the practises apart from the more traditional doctor/hospital methods most of us are familiar with.

Why do alternative healing?

Because the different modalities work to get to your unexpressed feelings, release them from your energy and bring balance to your system subsequently benefitting your physical body and the overall quality of your life.

Alternative healing methods encourage you to express, not suppress.

Listed here are some of the different methods of healing.

The most important thing to understand is that healing doesn't necessarily mean cure.

The best medicine in the world, alternative or otherwise, will not help you if, on some level, you don't truly wish it to. A surgeon can cut a disease from your body but if you don't make a change on an energy level, chances are the illness will return.

Each of the alternative healing methods described have their own merit and value. Which ones you choose are entirely up to you.

NB: Where necessary, the following treatments should only be administered by qualified practitioners.

Acupuncture

Originated in China over 5000 years ago. Selected points along the energy meridians of the body are stimulated by needles to remove blockages, improve and enhance the flow of ch'i and restore balance to the functioning of the internal organs of the body. Acupuncture can assist in the treatment of many ailments and is also used for the relief of pain.

Acupressure

Works on the exact same principle as acupuncture but rather than using needles to stimulate the flow of ch'i, finger pressure is applied to the acupuncture points. Reflexology of the hands and feet is done using acupressure.

Aromatherapy

Basically means 'a therapy using aromas'. It is the use of essential oils to heal body, mind and spirit. The oils are extracted from various parts of a plant, whether it be the petals, peel, leaves, wood, berries, seeds, or roots. The extraction process is very specific and is done in such a way so as to ensure the oils retain their therapeutic properties.

One of the main reasons the oils are so powerful is the link between your sense of smell and your emotions. At this level the oils can work to calm, balance or uplift you. On a physical level many of the oils have antiviral and antibacterial properties. Some of the uses of the oils, which can be used successfully alone or combined, are:

My choices always benefit me

- compresses
- in the bath
- in a massage oil
- for inhalations and vaporisation.

There are at least eighty essential oils available and some of the more common oils are basil, bergamot, chamomile, geranium, jasmine, lavender, patchouli, rosemary and tea tree. The benefits of aromatherapy are being recognised more and more and there are many excellent books which deal with the subject exclusively.

Bach Flower Remedies

This system of healing came into being in the 1930s and was the inspiration of an English physician - Dr. Edward Bach. Dr. Bach was highly intuitive and he felt that a person's personality impacted on their health so he concentrated his efforts on developing natural remedies for particular mood states or personality traits. Flower remedies are a vibrational therapy that work on an energy level to heal the emotional and spiritual causes of illness and re-establish balance on all levels.

At an address given in Southport in 1931, Dr. Bach said:

> "...the action of these remedies is to raise our vibrations and open up our channels for the reception of the spiritual self; to flood one's nature with the particular virtue we need and wash out from us the fault that is causing the harm."
> *(Howard and Ramsell, eds. 1990)*

In all, there are thirty eight different extracts which cover the entire range of human emotions. For instance, if you were suffering from persistent worrying thoughts you would take 'White Chestnut'. The remedies, which are completely natural and safe, are taken orally, either a couple of drops under the tongue or diluted in water or fruit juice.

Australian Bush Flower Remedies

Developed by naturopath Ian White, these remedies tap into the healing power of native Australian plants. There are over 60 essences including: Sunshine Wattle, Yellow Cowslip Orchid, Pink Mulla Mulla, Kangaroo Paw and She Oak. She Oak, for example, can be used to help women going through menopause as it balances the hormones. The remedies work in the same way as the Bach Flowers and Ian White has written several books on the unique essences.

Biochemic Tissue Salts

The human body is made up of an infinite number of cells and Dr. W. H. Schuessler, a 19th century physicist and physiological chemist, identified twelve individual 'tissue salts' within every cell. He determined that each of these tissue, or cell, salts was an essential mineral component of the body which aided the natural ability to make, and preserve, these level of cells. If the body was lacking in any of these mineral salts, loss of health occurred. If your cells were deficient in magnesium phosphate, for example, you might suffer from muscular cramps, spasms and minor nerve problems. Dr. Schuessler ascertained that if the deficiency was corrected, the body was able to heal itself. The tissue salts are prepared homoeopathically. This way the body is able to quickly and easily assimilate the minerals into the cells so the natural balance of the body is rapidly restored.

Bowen Therapy

Was developed in Australia by Tom Bowen. The treatment consists of a series of light, gentle movements over muscles, tendons and connective tissues applied in a precise sequence at specific points on the body. After the therapist has administered three or four of these movements the client is allowed to rest, giving the body time to absorb them before the next sequence is applied. No force is used or needed and the therapy encourages the body to relax and make the subtle adjustments needed to restore itself to a state of balance.

Breathwork and Rebirthing

By the use of breathing techniques, which tap into the emotions you're carrying around, breathwork and rebirthing work towards releasing blocked energies from the body. Both methods can be used quite separately but we'll discuss the two together as they share a similar purpose.

Breathwork and rebirthing are like a thorough spring clean.

Deep breathing helps to stir up the old, gluey, stagnant energies in your system, causing them to break down and dissipate, leaving you lighter and clearer so energy can once again flow freely. The freer the movement of energy, the healthier you are.

The breathing techniques used take you beyond your ordinary state of consciousness and in this way connect you to the deepest parts of your inner world. You become more in touch with the real you.

During a session you will breathe very deeply using a technique called 'Connected Breathing' which draws abundant energy and oxygen into your cells. You may experience sensations, emotions, pictures, or sounds that have been held and buried inside for a very long time.

As these surface, your body is allowed to express these emotions in a safe and nurturing environment guided by an experienced practitioner. After the feelings have been expressed, there is usually a feeling of release, peace and clarity.

This is a very personal and individual experience and releasing the blocks held in your body breaks down the barriers that hinder personal growth and the fulfilment of being all that you can be.

Chiropractic

Is a therapeutic system of treating conditions and curing ailments primarily through hands-on manipulation and adjustment of the spine and other joints. Chiropractors regard the body's nervous system as essential to good health and that all disease is traceable to nervous malfunctions usually caused by vertebrae that are misaligned.

The purpose of spinal adjustment is to relieve pressure on nerves thereby restoring balance to the body and its systems.

Crystals

Natural crystals are formed by minerals which are found in the Earth's crust. There are many different types of crystals and each type has its own structure and purpose. All crystals can be used in healing because they have the power to receive and transmit energy. Quartz crystal was initially used to transmit radio waves because of its ability to generate an electrical charge and in recent years has been used in computers.

Crystals are wonderful for balancing the energies of the body, particularly when used on the chakras. Like the chakras, crystals come in many different colours and it has been found that crystals which match the colour of the chakra work well when healing and balancing. If you tune your energies into those of your crystals you will find that you can communicate with them. Everything has consciousness.

Crystals love to heal and they love to be appreciated. Their energy, because it comes directly from our living earth, is very alive and all living things respond to kindness. We could extol the virtues of crystals for hours but there are many excellent books which explain the value and use of crystals in greater depth. Sharing your space with a crystal, or as many crystals as you desire, is one of the best things you can do for yourself.

Herbal Medicine

Herbs are the oldest form of medicine and the use of herbs for treating disease has been an integral part of the healing tradition of many cultures for thousands of years.

The recent growing concerns regarding the side effects of modern drugs has brought about a resurgence in herbal remedies. The properties of herbs are as many and varied as the herbs themselves and the subject is so broad that it would be a good idea to obtain some of the many excellent books that are available which deal exclusively with the subject.

Herbs are a powerful healing tool and well worth your time and attention but to attempt herbal medicine without assistance is not advisable. An overuse of some herbs can be toxic so it is important to study the use of herbs and even seek guidance from a qualified herbalist before using them.

Homoeopathy

Was first developed by a German doctor, Samuel Hahnemann, in 1796. It works on the premise that 'like cures like', meaning that a substance that can produce symptoms of illness in a well person can, in minute doses, cure similar symptoms of disease. It is believed that the body's immune system is stimulated by the introduction of the foreign substance. Some of the most powerful remedies are so diluted that they are actually operating on an energetic level rather than a chemical level, holding the 'memory' of the original substance. Homoeopaths prescribe treatment based on an in-depth, individual consultation whereby a remedy is chosen that matches an individual's needs.

Hypnotherapy

Hypnosis is a trance like state that resembles sleep and is induced by suggestion. In this highly relaxed state the subconscious mind is more easily accessed because the resistance of the conscious mind is bypassed. The subconscious mind holds onto everything you have experienced, whether you want it to or not.

What you carry around in your subconscious directly influences your behaviour and responses even though you're not aware of it. Hypnotherapy helps you access and release those things that have been suppressed which have a detrimental effect on your well-being.

The highly relaxed state that is induced by the therapist enables you to become susceptible to suggestions which are used to help you overcome addictions, anxiety and phobias, to manage pain, or enhance the healing of a variety of ailments.

Kinesiology

'Muscle testing' is the fundamental and key technique used in kinesiology. It has proved to be a remarkable tool for detecting and correcting imbalances in the body which may relate to stress, illness, nutrition, food intolerance, allergies, learning, traumatic past memories and even energy flow through the meridians.

Through the use of muscle testing, kinesiology uses the subconscious communication system of the body to identify the causes of imbalance. The techniques of kinesiology are applied to deal with the subtle, but many, imbalances that lie behind the physical, mental, emotional and spiritual problems that many people experience. Once the underlying cause of the issue has been determined, the body is then re-balanced.

Magnetic Therapy

Involves the use of magnetic force fields to treat back pain and other conditions. The force field is said to encourage muscle relaxation and blood flow which enables greater distribution of oxygen, promoting faster healing. Magnetic therapy is a good example of atoms at play. Without getting too complicated, magnetic forces are produced by the motion of charged particles, such as electrons. When a magnetic field is built up, these fields influence charged particles that move through them. As your entire body is made up of charged particles the magnets are, possibly, influencing your energy somehow and altering its condition at the atomic level.

How a magnet works is not entirely known, but results have shown that they just do. Research in this area is still continuing.

Massage

Is an ancient, intuitive form of healing body, mind and spirit. The essence of massage is a loving, caring touch which enhances the body's innate healing powers. There are a variety of basic strokes used in massage designed to bring about certain physiological and psychological effects in the body and mind.

From a physiological point of view, massage promotes the flow of blood and lymph towards the heart, increasing oxygen and nutrients in the cells, eliminating body wastes and excess fluid and stimulating the immune system. The soothing strokes sedate and relax the whole central nervous system making more energy available to the body.

I feel my connection to nature

Massage also helps to free restricted nerve roots. Hard, contracted muscles are stretched and softened and hard knots can be released. Chronically relaxed muscles are toned and strengthened.

When muscles are functioning as they should be, the skeleton and its joints maintain balance and position. Massage also enhances the activity of the digestive, endocrine and respiratory systems and nourishes and conditions the skin.

Psychologically, massage gives you a sense of comfort and well-being, one of the reasons being that it encourages the production of endorphins. Being touched in a loving way satisfies emotional needs for caring and nurturing. The mind is relaxed and emotional tension is relieved.

From an energetic perspective, massage aids in the continuous and harmonious flow of ch'i energies. Massage and bodywork also create for you a greater awareness of your own body and its communication to you.

Naturopathy

Translates as 'natural treatment'. Many naturopaths believe that the four basic components of good health are clean air, clean water, clean food from good soil and exercise. "Right living" is encouraged. Symptoms of illness are a sign that the body is out of balance and attempting to eliminate toxins. Naturopathic medicine uses a variety of natural, non-toxic therapies and treatments in an effort to cleanse the body. One of the main principles of naturopathy is that the body has the power to heal itself and treatment, which is prescribed on a wholistic basis, is given to support this process.

Reiki

Pronounced Ray-Key - is a Japanese word meaning 'Universal Life Energy' and is an ancient method of energy healing. It is a form of energy which is channelled from the Universe, through the healer and into the recipient via the laying on of hands. Reiki energy can also be 'sent' to a person or situation. This is referred to as absent healing.

The essence of Reiki is a pure and loving energy. To use Reiki in healing, the healer is 'attuned' to the universal life force by a Reiki Master. This then expands the ability to tap into the energy. Reiki is predominantly a healing energy but it is never sent or forced into the body. Rather, it is taken in by the person, or the animal, according to how much they're willing to accept.

During a Reiki session the recipient usually experiences deep relaxation. An increased flow of energy and vitality may follow the session. Anyone can be attuned to Reiki and you can use it to heal yourself as well as others.

Reflexology

The practise of reflexology goes back some four thousand years to ancient China and is performed on the feet and hands. All areas of the feet and hands mirror different organs, glands and body parts. Massaging and applying pressure to these areas stimulates and strengthens the corresponding regions and promotes healing.

Reflexology is also effective in relieving tension and stress, improving circulation, cleansing toxins and revitalising energy. As the internal organs of your body are also associated with emotions such as fear, grief and anger, regular reflexology helps to bring balance to the body, mind and emotions.

Rolfing

Is named after its founder Dr. Ida Rolf (1896-1979), an American biochemist. Rolfing relies mainly on deep massage of the muscles and connective tissues (fascia). It involves various manipulations to stretch tight and thickened fascia that may be causing misalignment somewhere in the body. When this happens, the body compensates by making changes in another area, eventually weakening the entire structure.

The aim of the Rolfer is to realign the body structure to restore freedom, movement and balance. Emotional and physical problems may surface during the treatment, which usually involves a series of approximately ten hourly sessions.

Shiatsu

Is a healing art that originated in Japan and means 'finger massage'. Shiatsu practitioners use not only their fingers but other parts of their bodies such as thumbs, elbows, knees and feet to apply pressure to stimulate the flow of energy through the meridians for health and well-being.

Shiatsu is different to massage in that there are no smooth, flowing strokes, no kneading or friction and no use of oils. The patient remains fully clothed whilst treatment is administered. Traditional shiatsu is usually performed on a futon.

Shiatsu is beneficial in many ways. It helps to release deep emotional issues, encourages balance and relaxation, reduces stress, is calming to the nervous system, boosts stamina, improves body functions such as digestion, and relieves pain.

The healing that shiatsu provides, balances the body as a whole rather than treating specific ailments.

Somatic Movement

The word 'somatic' comes from the Greek word 'soma' meaning body.

Somatic movement is about connecting to your body and being aware and present during the movement. This assists people to release built up emotions and old traumas held in the body and reduce physical tension.

Movements such as shaking or rocking encourage the body to release, thus allowing energy to flow.

Sound Therapy

Is the directing of sound waves, at specific frequencies, to influence the vibration of a particular body part therefore restoring balance and, ultimately, health. Like Magnetic Therapy, sound therapy most likely works at an atomic level because your energy responds to the resonance of sound. For instance, loud noise can set nerves on edge; soft music can relax; screams can upset.

The bulk of the human body is made up of water and

sound travels faster through water than air. This may well be a factor in the body's ability to respond to the molecular make-up of sound. When the subtle energies in a particular area of the human body have been disrupted, the sound waves may be resonating with the molecules within that area thereby altering the state of the energy bringing it back to its correct vibrational rate.

Trager

Created by Chicago physician Dr. Milton Trager to help victims of polio and various neuromuscular disorders. It involves a combination of light massage strokes with gentle, rhythmic bouncing, shaking and rocking movements of the trunk and limbs to promote real flexibility of limb motion. Clients are encouraged to relax deeply to bypass the muscular control of the conscious mind and allow the unconscious mind to accept and integrate the freer, less restrictive body movements as demonstrated by the practitioner. Clients are then given some instruction in the use of mentastics, a system of simple, mind-directed movements they practice at home between sessions to keep the body flexible and pain-free.

Aura, Chakra and Spiritual Healing

Your aura and chakras are part of your spiritual system which is comprised purely of energy. The healing and balancing of these energies can be collectively termed 'spiritual healing'. Basically, the healer sets the vibrational tone that you need to match to bring about balance. It is you who has the power to choose. Another person cannot actually 'heal' you.

Energy healing benefits your overall health because illness begins on an energy level and will ultimately manifest in the body if any imbalances are not addressed. Through a healer, vital energy is channelled from the spiritual source. It then flows through their hands and into the recipient. The healer may lay hands on the physical body or work only on the energy fields surrounding the body.

In spiritual healing, positive energies
supplant negative energies.

When we refer to positive and negative energies we're not talking about energies that are 'good' and 'bad'. With negative energy we're talking about energy that causes imbalances - blocked, stagnant masses that hinder the natural flow of your body's energy. Positive energy is new, vital, healing and cleansing.

Earlier we discussed the composition of your aura and chakras and some of the issues relevant to them. Here we'll look at some of the more common ways in which they are affected by health and how they can be healed and balanced.

We know the energy of your aura and chakras
is sensitive to the conditions of your
mental and emotional health.

Within your aura and chakras you can manifest blockages, weaknesses, rips, tears, imbalances, stagnation and a general disruption and depletion of the smooth flow of energy. Some of the ways in which these things can be caused are:

- the stresses of day to day living
- old traumas and injuries
- self-destructive beliefs and patterns of behaviour
- unresolved emotional issues
- fears
- negative thoughts and words directed at the self and others
- suppressed feelings
- drugs, alcohol and smoking

Not only are you capable of hindering the flow of energy you can also build up what is known as 'energetic armour'.

The armour serves to act as a defence system and by setting up this shielding you aim to protect yourself from feeling insecure, vulnerable, emotionally threatened, or unsafe. Additionally it helps you to avoid confronting your true feelings and eventually you are able to numb them.

You might think you're escaping your emotions by setting up barriers but because your energy doesn't understand about the concept of denial it leaves you with physical indicators that something is amiss.

Armour will show up in the body as an area of high tension and muscle tightness or you may develop excessive muscle, fat, or bloating around the parts where the armour sits.

Any of these things around the torso area, for instance, may be an indication that you are emotionally shielding your sacral, solar plexus and/or heart chakra regions.

*The job of your chakras is to attract
the universal life-force energy.*

It is drawn into, and moved throughout, your physical body and auric field by your chakra network. The energy taken in directly influences the workings of your entire body systems. This is why it's important for these systems to be healthy so the new energy that's always coming in can benefit you in the ways it's supposed to.

*If you have blockages in your energy fields,
it becomes hard for the incoming energy to
penetrate the blocks and dissolve them.*

Repairs to tears and holes becomes more difficult also as energy tends to flow straight out of them.

Healing performed on your aura and chakras works to repair, cleanse, balance and revitalise these energy fields. New energy that holds light or colour is brought in to replace any energy the healer may extract.

Here is a general idea of what may occur during a typical healing session.

The healer, who acts as a conduit for universal and spiritual energy, has agreed to be a clear and open channel for the healing energies to flow through her/him. Using intuition, psychic perception and spiritual guidance, the healer analyses the patient's energy systems and senses, or sees, any blockages or imbalances in the flow of energy.

A healer may perceive these energies as being heavy, dark, or sticky.

Oils: Lemon for Purification

Before beginning, the healer connects to the highest energies of love and light and sets a clear intention for the purpose of the healing.

Usually the intention is that the healing being administered be for the highest good of the patient. The request is a simple one because a healer never attaches a personal desire as to how s/he would like a healing to progress. Instead, the healer's 'Will' aligns with 'Divine Will' and trusts that what is needed to be done, will be done.

From a spiritual perspective much more is known about what a patient truly desires and requires.

With no specific outcome for the session in mind the healer then sets about cleansing and charging the aura and chakras with healing energy.

In relation to the aura, some areas may have an excess of energy and other areas may be deficient. Usually areas of high tension, such as the shoulders, neck and head tend to develop excessive energy deposits. Tears, leaks, holes and even loss of colour within the aura are indicative that the life-force energy is draining away and when this is happening the person is usually feeling very weak on more levels than just the physical.

The healer works to smooth and repair the energies, clear blocks, stabilise the fields and redistribute the energy evenly, restoring balance.

Energy that is directed into the chakras will begin to break down blockages. At this point, as they're being opened up and cleared, it's quite usual for unresolved emotional issues to begin surfacing. Psychologically, lessons relating to the chakras will come into the patient's awareness also.

The patient is encouraged to breathe deeply and to feel and express whatever comes up.

A release, such as crying, may occur. The healer may then be further guided to cleanse and clear other areas and do any repairs that are needed. The energetic fields are then balanced, smoothed and calmed.

Crystals may be used to assist with the healing.

Negative energy is a very real thing and it not only needs to be removed from the body, it also needs to be recycled back into a positive state. The healer assists this process by loosening the blocked energy and using her/his hands to scoop or lift it out of the body.

This energy is usually handed to spirit guides with the intention that it be replenished and revitalised or turned into white light. It is not just carelessly dumped in the room somewhere or into anybody's energy field. It is always handled responsibly.

During a healing, it's important for the patient to work in conjunction with the healer in the respect of also setting an intention for what they desire to gain from the healing and then being willing to acknowledge and release blocks.

Current and limiting belief systems must be challenged if the patient is to heal and, therefore, change.

This is imperative so as not to manifest other blockages or imbalances in place of any that have just been cleared. If change doesn't take place on an emotional level, the same problems will continue to occur.

The wonderful thing about energy is that it will always flow to where it is needed the most and self-healing is possible.

You can work on your aura and chakras by:

- sending loving energy in and out of your heart chakra
- laying on of your own hands and asking for the healing, spiritual energy to flow through you
- giving yourself Reiki
- visualising being surrounded by healing energies
- breathing deeply to stir up sluggish energy
- using aromatherapy oils, meditation, colour, sound
- repeating affirmations
- releasing and resolving emotional issues
- raising your vibration through the practise of gratitude and appreciation

Like the immune system of your physical body your energy systems also work to heal themselves but blockages may hinder this. Fortunately, the laying on of hands accelerates and enhances the healing process.

A healing touch boosts your body's innate healing forces.

With any form of healing you will make your own decision as to how much healing you'll accept. This also applies in absent healing or when projecting energy, love and light. Healers never ask for a specific result and always leave the outcome to the higher forces. Only your higher self knows what is best for you.

Love is the force that motivates all healers.

Recommended Reading

There is a diverse amount of material in this book and what we have given you is a starting point from which to go by. It's an interesting world that lies beyond your five physical senses so we highly recommend that you delve deeper into all the areas that interest you. There is a large range of specialised information available.

Below is a list of authors who are well worth reading.

There are many, many more wonderful authors who could have easily been added to the list but you will undoubtedly find them yourself (or they will 'find' you).

Richard Bach	Dr. Elisabeth Kübler-Ross
Daryl Anka-Bashar	Dr Nicole LePera
Brandon Bays	Harriet Goldhor Lerner
Barbara Ann Brennan	Caroline M. Myss
Deepak Chopra	Michael Newton
Paulo Coelho - The Alchemist	M. Scott Peck
Dr. Wayne W. Dyer	James Redfield
Shakti Gawain	Jane Roberts - Seth books
Edmund Harold	Sanaya Roman
Louise L. Hay	Inna Segal
Esther & Jerry Hicks - Abraham	Shefali Tsabary
Dawn Hill	Joe Vitale
Soozi Holbeche	Neale Donald Walsch
Susan Jeffers	Stuart Wilde
Karen Kingston	Marianne Williamson

Other resources: 'Better Blended' eBook by Lauren Saliu - payhip.com/laurensaliu

May your journey be rewarding, fulfilling and meaningful.

Blessed Be.

Reference List

Brennan, Barbara Ann. Hands of Light. Bantam Books, New York, 1987.

Bach, E. (1931) Ye Suffer from Yourselves. In Howard, J. and Ramsell, J. eds. (1990) Original Writings of Edward Bach, p. 62, Saffron Walden, C. W. Daniel.

www.ingramcontent.com/pod-product-compliance
Lightning Source LLC
Chambersburg PA
CBHW061656040426
42446CB00010B/1760